# Detox Cleanse Your Body Quickly and Completely

Bill Bodri

Top Shape Publishing LLC
1135 Terminal Way Suite 209
Reno, NV 89502


ISBN-10: 0-9980764-4-9
ISBN-13: 978-0-9980764-4-7

# DISCLAIMER

The information contained in this book (and any accompanying material) is intended for educational purposes only and is not intended to replace the attention, advice or care of a physician or other qualified health care professional. It has not been reviewed or approved by the FDA. It is not meant to cover all possible precautions, drug interactions, circumstances or adverse effects. Anyone who wishes to embark on any dietary, drug, exercise, or other lifestyle change intended to detox the body or prevent or treat a specific disease or condition should first consult with and seek clearance from a physician or other qualified health care professional. You should seek prompt medical care for any health issues and consult your doctor before using any of these protocols or making a change to your health regimen. Pregnant women in particular should seek the advice of a physician before using any protocols in this book. The protocols described are for adults only, unless otherwise specified. Product labels may contain important safety information and the most recent product information provided by the product manufacturers should be carefully reviewed prior to use to verify the dose, administration, and contraindications. National, state, and local laws may vary regarding the use and application of many of the treatments discussed. The reader assumes the risk of any injuries. The authors and publishers, their affiliates and assigns are not liable for any injury and/or damage to persons arising from this protocol and expressly disclaim responsibility for any adverse effects resulting from the use of the information contained herein. The protocols raise many issues that are subject to change as new data emerge. None of the suggested protocol regimens can guarantee health benefits. The publisher has not performed independent verification of the data contained herein, and expressly disclaim responsibility for any error in literature.

BILL BODRI

# CONTENTS

# ACKNOWLEDGMENTS

This book would never have been possible without my introduction to the nutritional and detoxification teachings of Edgar Cayce, Bernard Jenson, Dr. Jonathan Wright, Dr. Julian Whitaker, Dr. David Williams, Dr. Dietrich Klinghardt, Dr. Joseph Mercola, Doc Wheelright, John Christopher, Richard Schulze, Gary Null, Jeffrey Bland, Burton Goldberg, David Getoff and an entire host of alternative physicians too numerous to mention as well as the Rodale Press, Acres USA and the Price-Pottenger Foundation.

# 1
## INTRODUCTION

As a nutritionist I hear lots of sorrowful stories of health problems where the doctors just haven't been able to help their patients. Some people tell me they are fighting a terrible sickness or disease and are seeking any help possible beyond what standard medicine has to offer. Many have told me they have tried everything and they don't know what to do anymore.

Nutritionists like me also encounter quite a few people seeking to lose weight after trying countless diets and failing. One common weight loss issue is that some individuals will begin to lose weight, start to feel terrible and then quit. They don't know that their body stores toxins in its fat tissues so that when they lose weight those toxins are released into their bloodstream, thus producing the feelings of unease. They would be much more successful at weight loss if they started with several rounds of detoxification first.

Rare it is that people come to me without any specific health issue and tell me they simply want to look and feel better. Those individuals are the smart ones, however, because they are practicing prevention. Those wise ones usually ask me about any new "miracle" supplements on the market they have heard about and the minimum they can do to get the greatest help for the least amount of effort in terms of general anti-aging and health improvement.

Undertaking a detoxification program at home can often help with all these issues. It is one of the single most important things you can do for your health because it will cleanse your body of conditions that cause aging and disease. Often it will reduce your sensitivities and decrease your risks of cancer or other illnesses. A detox program can help you lose weight, discharge toxins and poisons from the body so that you look younger and feel better, and by cleansing your body can often help cure disease. An effective detox program can be life-changing.

One problem with the world today is that it has become terribly polluted and we are absorbing this pollution. Being exposed to toxic chemicals in the air, our water and food, over time our bodies have silently absorbed an innumerable bevy of harmful contaminants including heavy metals (such as lead, mercury, cadmium, and aluminum), insecticide and pesticide remnants, xenoestrogens, plastics, toxic chemicals, inoculation residues, and many other poisons – all of which have collected in the cells of our muscles, blood, lymphatic fluid and cerebral spinal fluid. Because of this accumulated onslaught our bodies have become a toxic cesspool.

We are all suffering from a lifetime accumulation of chemicals ingested from our food, water and the air we breath because our liver, kidneys and other detoxification organs have not been able to keep up with the incredible deluge to eliminate them. Detoxification tries to get rid of this accumulated filth so that the body's workings can become normalized once again.

In a 2002 landmark study performed by the Environmental Working Group (EWG), nine Americans who did not work with chemicals in their jobs were tested for 210 different toxic chemicals associated with human health problems. A total of 167 toxic chemicals were found in the nine participants, each showing an average of 91 harmful chemical in their body. In a later study also spearheaded by the EWG, an average of 200 industrial compounds, pollutants and other chemicals were found in 10 newborn babies with 287 different chemicals being discovered in total.

This astounding amount of toxic chemical residues is what you can now expect to find in an average American infant! We are all being polluted, and if this continues we might have to finish that statement with "polluted to death." Of those 287 chemicals found in infants, science knows that 180 cause cancer, 217 are toxic to the brain or nervous system, and 208 cause developmental problems. We have poisoned the planet and now those poisons are finding a home within us. Detoxification is the only way to reduce the harmful effects of this new internal burden.

EPA studies also show that 100% of people now have harmful PCBs, dioxins, xylene, dichlorobenzene and other harmful chemicals stored in their fat cells. Studies of human breathing additionally indicate harmful chemicals being released from our breath such as carcinogenic benzene and perchloroethylene in 89% and 93% of cases respectively. Don't you think that these chemicals, stored inside us, are interfering with our natural biological processes and contributing to disease? They are. They help cause disease.

This internal accumulation can only be countered by periodic detoxification efforts you must undertake yourself. If you want to look better and feel better and reduce your risks of cancer and other debilitating diseases you should periodically do something to help your body get rid of accumulated toxic stores. You must also nutritionally support your own organs of detoxification.

Anyone could easily bring up dozens of studies that basically make the same point that all of us have accumulated so many unwanted toxins in our bodies that they now stand behind the onset of many diseases and physical malfunctions. Toxic accumulations within your body, such as heavy metals, are often responsible for the mysterious symptoms people suffer from that baffle doctors.

The solution to a healthier you is to detoxify your body and its organs of as many types of chemical accumulations as possible - heavy metals, toxins, plaque, pesticides, and chemicals. You need to work on detoxifying your skin, bones, intestines, kidneys, liver and other tissues of harmful accumulations which are there since your body stored them away in cells when it could not keep up with the task of removing them. Different people will require different products for their own detoxification needs, but a typical protocol will be to start with the intestines, kidneys and liver since they are our main detoxifiers or channels of elimination. Those three organs are the major detoxification trio. Once you strengthen these organs and detox them enough that they start cleansing and healing themselves, then you can proceed onto a deeper level of detox effort.

Detoxification regimens can run from the totally useless to the highly beneficial. I only want to communicate to you what I consider the best, but also the simplest for getting started. For many years, health care professionals have been trying out various natural substances and protocols in an attempt to effectively cleanse their patients' bodies of all these pollutant chemicals, always attempting to increase their success and reduce the possible side effects. Their goal has been to cure disease, increase their patients' health and energy, restore functionality and extend their lifespans.

Inside you will find a collection of some of the most powerful detoxification protocols you can do at home using products that others have derived from years of development. I've left out most detoxification diet discussions since that is an entire topic in itself and basically comes down to *eating nutritionally dense clean food*. Most people who come to me just want to get started with a detox effort and are unwilling to yet make major changes in their diet (until they are really in trouble), so we will be focusing in on just basic detoxification efforts alone. For the best dietary advice anyone can provide, I would like to direct you to the Price-Pottenger Foundation.

Most detoxification programs do not "chelate," meaning remove metal and chemical toxins from the body. Rather, they optimize your body's internal detoxification mechanisms so that they can do a better job of getting rid of wastes. However, inside you will find chelation protocols as well that actually grab unwanted toxins and help escort them out of your body. However, your first priority should be to get your channels of detoxification working, and only afterwards should you go full blast with countless detoxifiers to help your body go into a multi-month or multi-year detox mode. If you want to do it correctly, it will take a minimum of over a year to really and truly detox your body completely.

In the field of human biochemistry, detoxification involves a series of enzymatic reactions that neutralize and solubilize toxins, and then transports them to eliminatory organs such as the liver or kidneys so they can be excreted from the body through the stool or urine. Cellular detoxification actively releases toxins from the tissues and organs of the body into the blood stream, so on some level it is equivalent to continuously poisoning the body if those toxins are not eventually eliminated from your system. Since that is the case, you must be careful not to try to detox too quickly or you will land in a heap of trouble. You might overwhelm your detox organs by releasing too many poisons into your system that you are unprepared to handle.

As stated, the problem is now that the onslaught of toxins in today's polluted world has become so severe that the body's detoxification systems have not been able to keep pace with the demand for their services. Thus, most people have found that excess toxins have started accumulating in their body and started contributing to weight loss issues, sickness, aging and disease. The end result is that people don't look as good as they once did, cannot do as much as they once could, and don't feel as well either.

A home detoxification program is the remedy. However, a detoxification regime will usually tax your organs of elimination since they are probably already under strain. Because of that strain, once again I want to issue the warning that it is important not to try to detox too much all at once. Overdoing it by trying too many things at the same time may exceed your detoxification capacity and then you will be poisoning yourself to some degree until the toxins are cleared out of your system. This will manifest through headaches, irritation, skin eruptions, sleeplessness, fatigue and other uncomfortable symptoms. You won't feel well if you try to rush it.

Whenever you put an additional burden on your detoxification organs you must also take supportive nutrients so that your liver and kidney have enough energy to carry out the additional work you are requesting of them. Over time, cellular detoxification will tend to deplete the energy and nutrient reserves of these organs so you must ingest supportive nutrients geared to each organ. This will ensure that the energetic levels and general function of these organs can accommodate your current level of detoxification and elimination. This is why conservatively pacing yourself, and taking regular breaks in your detoxification schedule, are very important.

Remember that detoxification focuses on eliminating toxic substances and pulling them out of your body through its normal detoxification pathways. This requires that you support all of the systems of your body to encourage its own natural cleansing abilities. Using supplements it would be wise to support the body's own ability to cleanse itself during a detox program so that it can purge itself of the toxins that have been accumulated.

When you want to detoxify your body, I feel that one of the best places to start – since it is one of the easiest tasks to accomplish - is by first working on your colon and intestines to get them moving and fully expelling wastes. Once you have gotten rid of any constipation issues and eliminated intestinal micro-organisms such as parasites, bacteria, yeast and fungus you can then start working on removing poisons from your body. After the toxic burden within subsides because of your detoxification efforts you can work on building up your health again.

Therefore after getting the colon and intestines moving, the next part of a detoxification regime should focus on removing poisons from throughout your body. The priority is to then focus on your liver and kidneys, and next the connective tissues and other organs of your body as need be. After you detox an organ you can then focus on supporting or building it back up again without the presence of poisons that might interfere with recovery.

There are detoxification protocols inside provided for various parts of the body, but many people just want something simple that works on everything at the same time. Therefore we will start with the detoxification program I do every year for myself, which is one of the simplest but most powerful of the many all-body protocols I have encountered over the years. People always ask me for something simple they can follow 1-2-3 and this is it.

You can purchase fantastic multi-month detoxification kits with many ingredients, such as the excellent detoxification kit from Systemic Formulas, but most people tell me they just want to start with something simple. Therefore this is where we are going to start.

2

# A SIMPLE BASIC DETOX PROGRAM

As a nutritionist who helps people with their health problems, I get a lot of questions about how to detox and support the body when it doesn't seem to be working as well as it used to when people were younger. Those questions caused me to develop a series of very successful detoxification retreats in Asia where we would start people on their way to internal cleansing and help them address some basic health issues.

Most people don't have time for a detoxification retreat, but they still want a simple all-body detox program to help get rid of the accumulated chemicals and wastes in their body that have built up over the years. They are also hoping to possibly help solve some long-standing health issues because they heard that detoxification can often do this. They don't want to spend time with a professional who will help them slowly but safely detoxify chemicals from their body. They tell me they just want some simple things they can do on their own, without getting too complicated, so that they can get started.

It is not surprising that one of the most common questions I heard from these individuals was, "What is the simplest, cheapest but most effective detox program I can use that employs the fewest supplements but gets great results?"

The answer I typically gave is based upon a protocol I first learned from superstar naturopath David Getoff many years ago. I have found that this small set of detoxification supplements he recommended, which uses "just three bottles of pills," is gentle

7

enough for most people to handle, starts showing results in a very short period of time, and works wonders for most everyone.

Many people will start feeling more energy, sleep better, lose weight, experience a general improvement in mood, and dramatically improve the appearance of their skin after they start using these three detoxification products in tandem, which constitute my fundamental detox routine and the program I use myself once per year. The basic supplements are:

Nature's Pure Body Whole Body Program & Colon Program
  (Pure Body Institute)
Vitalzym (World Nutrition)

Just these three detoxification products alone, taken together, will start making you look and feel younger. I usually add a kidney flush to this mix, using Dr. Schulze's K-B (Kidney-Bladder) Tea, but these three products (Vitalzym and the Nature's Whole Body Program and Colon Cleanse) constitute my fundamental detox routine for people who want to start making a dent in removing chemicals and toxins from their body, do not have the help of a knowledgeable practitioner available but want to proceed safely, and do not want to use too much time, money or effort.

The Nature's Pure Body Whole Body Program and Colon Cleanse contains two different bottles of herbal supplements that remove wastes at the cellular level in your body. They are not herbal supplements that "send in agents" to pull out toxins, so they don't actively force cellular cleansing as is done through chelation therapy. Their inventor told me that they won't pull toxins out of the tissues, but your body will release toxins as it slowly becomes healthier from their usage and improves its ability to eliminate wastes. The Whole Body Program tends to cleanse cellular wastes from your connective tissues while the Colon Program helps to make sure your intestines are eliminating the toxins being released.

What first attracted me to the Whole Body Program is a published study I read years ago in some nutritional journal showing that it was measuring the poisons and toxic materials eliminated from the body due to various detox products, and this product was the clear winner. One naturopath who also extensively uses the products told me he does so because they are the most dependable for producing dramatic improvements in people's health. Together with a scientist the two tried to figure out why the products were working so well and reasoned that they are freeing up the CoQ10 inside cells which spark energy production. If the CoQ10 within cells no longer has to be preoccupied with removing cellular wastes then the cells can devote their energies to DNA/RNA repair mechanisms, which may explain why the products get great results. This is also an argument for detoxification in general.

Vitalzym, on the other hand, works by helping to dissolve fibrin deposits in your body, break down micro-organism biofilms in your GI tract, and cleave toxins floating in your blood. This is a product that will eat away at post-operative scar tissue in your body because it will work on dissolving fibrin, but I basically think of it as a blood cleaner even though it gets busy at breaking down old diseased body tissues. As a collection of enzymes, Vitalzym basically dissolves problems that have accumulated within you over time. It can also be used to reduce inflammation caused by sprains and strains, and over time may improve quite a few health conditions.

Vitalzym contains a set of proteolytic enzymes (serrapeptase, bromelain, amylase, amla, lipase, protease, rutin, papain) designed to support health and counter any growing fibrosis within your organs. Use the manufacturing instructions on the bottle to find your activation dose, but know that a common long-term way to use it is to take 3 capsules twice a day for about a year.

When you first start using Vitalzym it will begin to remove excess fibrin from your organs and tissues, and the reaction might be a bit strong so that you can only increase the dosage slowly. As a blood cleanser it will also clear your blood of roaming toxins, breaking them down upon contact to support their detoxification and removal. Whereas you can feel and see the results of the Nature's Pure Body Program rather quickly, it usually takes weeks to notice significant changes from using Vitalzym. However, putting the two together is an effective way to work on detoxifying different systems of your body. The first few days of taking the products, however, requires some adjustment and can produce detoxification reactions.

If you experience cleansing reactions such as headaches or an upset stomach from using the Nature's Pure Body supplements, you should reduce the dosage of pills you are taking. For instance, you usually take 3 pills of the Nature's Pure Body and 1 pill of the Colon

Cleanse before breakfast and dinner. If you experience a headache at this rate then you are detoxing too fast and reabsorbing waste before elimination, so you should increase the Colon Cleanse from 1 to 2 capsules and cut back on the Whole Body Program from 3 to 2 capsules. You should also drink more water.

Vitalzym, on the other hand, may cause flu-like symptoms when it starts cleansing your blood. Some people might additionally feel a bit of nausea for the first few days they start taking the product, and you should cut down on the number of capsules taken if this happens. It is also possible to experience an increase in bowel movements, skin rashes or even headaches, which are all signs that detoxification is going on. Therefore you must gradually increase the dosage to avoid such symptoms.

The last part of a basic, simple detoxification trio is Dr. Schulze's K-B (Kidney-Bladder) Tea. A package of the K-B tea lasts about a week and its formulation is based upon herbs that help detoxify and drain your kidneys, which is very helpful when undergoing a detox routine. This is a tasty tea that doesn't add any burden to the body, so I like to use it at the same time I am using these other products. I have seen people eliminate long-standing kidney issues, urinary tract issues, migraine headaches and stubborn psoriasis just from one bag of K-B tea alone, although you should use more tea for a detox that lasts longer than one month.

Some people who have the money splurge for Dr. Schulze's 5-day Kidney-Bladder Detox kit that contains extra tinctures of kidney-bladder detox herbs, and this is a great addition to your detox program if you can afford it. A kit just makes things simple, but after one or two kits most people go for just the tea.

As a nutritionist I've tried hundreds of products over the years, and only use or recommend the ones I think are best. I'm not selling any of these products so I'm not making any money from them. I'm just telling you my experience of what works to give you the biggest (and safest) bang for your buck.

## Detoxification Exercise and Lymph Drainage

Since most people want to see the results of detoxification immediately start appearing as better skin, which is what quickly happens from this protocol, it is important to recommend exercise as another way to help cleanse your skin and connective tissues. What most people don't realize is that rebounders (mini trampolines), power plates, or pogo sticks are three of the best very ways to exercise to detoxify your skin and other tissues because all these forms of exercise shake every cell of your body simultaneously.

I love various forms of weight-bearing exercise, kettlebells, yoga and martial arts, but for detox I recommend these bouncy types of exercise in order to stimulate your lymphatic system since it is one of your body's main detoxification systems. As a form of detoxification no other exercise comes close to being bouncy. The major supplements I use for lymph congestion or to support lymphatic function are Apex Energetics TerrainMax Lymph Terrain, Herbalist & Alchemist Burdock/Red Root Compound, and Lymphomyosot by Heel.

Not only will rebounders, power plates or pogo sticks help with lymphatic drainage and detoxification but jumping for health is a more effective fitness exercise than running, jogging or cycling. It also produces fewer injuries. Rebound exercise strengthens every single cell of your body including those within your bones, cartilage, joints and all your body organs. It also helps improve digestion and rhythmical bowel activity. In other words, it helps relieve constipation by stimulating the muscular contractions of your colon, and this will prevent the reabsorption of wastes from a slow-moving bowel.

All your cells are stimulated and strengthened through the mechanics of bouncing up and down. The up and down motion compresses and decompresses your body's tissues and fluids to squeeze toxins out of the cells and tissues as lymph fluid is pushed through your body. Basically, toxins are washed out of tissues throughout the entire body and flushed out when you take up bouncing.

If you want to help loosen cellular debris for your detoxification efforts, as well as help your lymph system carry nutrients to every cell and carry waste products away, choose fun exercises that stimulate all your internal organs and move as many of your body cells as possible such as these.

## Eliminating Joint Pain

This brings up a final issue that I am asked about quite frequently at detoxification seminars. Most people who are interested in detoxification are older, and they usually complain of pain in their joints. Detoxification may help with this issue, but usually the problem has to be addressed another way.

Joint pain problems should be diagnosed by a doctor, but there is a nutritional product that is so inexpensive (usually around $10) that I often recommend people try it for various joint pains such as knee problems. That product is collagen (peptides) types 1 & 3 or collagen type 2.

Some people have told me that collagen powder cuts their pain in half within two days, and often I hear it completely cures people of joint pain in less than a week. You can buy collagen #1 and #3, or collagen #2, with my preferred brands being NeoCell, Jarrow or Sports Research Pure Collagen Peptides Powder.

Glucosamine is the other most commonly product for joint pain recommended by doctors, and the one I use is the Freeda brand of glucosamine, but without chondroitin sulfate since most people don't need it since they will build their own. If you buy a chondroitin sulfate product and you are not improving in five weeks time then you should stop spending the extra money for it.

There is another home remedy you can try for arthritis pain, especially the painful finger nodules that some people develop due to typing. That remedy is gin-soaked raisins. One of my previous bosses first introduced this remedy to me, which I had never heard of, after it produced a miraculous cure of his painful finger nodules over six months time. He, in turn, had been introduced to the remedy by a friend who had also used it to solve his finger arthritis problems.

To prepare the remedy you place a box of golden raisins in a jar or bowl, and then pour in gin made from juniper berries until the golden raisins are completely covered. You let the yellow raisins sit at room temperature for several days and soak up the gin. Cover the container with cheesecloth and let the raisins absorb the gin while the remaining liquid evaporates. After that you simply eat 10 or so raisins per day, which is about a spoonful.

Another pain-removing remedy for the joints is exercise specifically designed to rehabilitate joints. In my opinion, the best joint exercises in the world are "Z-Health" exercises based on circular movements to increase joint mobility. These simple exercises, which you can learn through a Z-Health DVD, take only about 10 minutes per day to perform. They slowly improve joint pains that people thought they would have forever.

One step removed from the joints is tendon health, and the best tendon stretching exercises I have found are Chinese *Yijin Jing* exercises, which can also be learned through videos.

Past the joints and tendons we come to muscles, and then we have exercise options like yoga and Pilates to stretch your muscles and tendons. There are also gym workouts and Activated Isolated Stretching exercises invented by Aaron Mattes. An inexpensive infrared (IR) light device such as the MedLight 630Pro can be used to help eliminate muscle sprains.

Going one step higher we have active movement exercises (rather than yoga) such as the soft martial arts of *Tai chi, Aikido, Xing Yi Quan* and *Baguazhang.* The soft martial arts are preferred over the hard martial arts, such as Judo and Karate, when you want to protect your joints from damage.

There are other types of exercises you can do to eliminate pains and get in shape, but I have focused on introducing the simplest and quickest types I know for removing pain (Z-Health for joints and *Yijin Jing* for tendons) to those requiring more time and commitment (Yoga, Pilates and the martial arts). If you want to get rid of joint pains, heal old injuries and increase joint flexibility, you can try supplements together with exercise to produce the result you want.

Reviewing, to start you didn't only get a simple detox program but also just received the simplest remedies I know to help eliminate (or should we say "detox") joint pain, which through experience appears to me to be a very common issue for those most interested in detoxification.

# 3
# COLON CLEANSING

We cannot talk about detoxification without addressing the issue of the colon and intestines since they excrete the majority of digestive and metabolic wastes from the body. In fact, for some people the word "detoxification" conjures up only one issue in their mind - how to get their colon working again to expel wastes more frequently. In other words, to many people detoxification means eliminating constipation.

Intestinal detoxification and healing actually entails addressing four major problems: (1) intestinal parasites, (2) Candida (yeast) infections, (3) constipation, and (4) intestinal permeability issues.

Constipation is the particularly troublesome issue of these four because it usually takes a lot of time to solve the problem permanently. Furthermore, dealing with constipation often requires testing a lot of different products or methods to see what works and those adjustments take time.

Handling Candida yeast and fungus overgrowth is also an issue that takes time to fix, like constipation, because in addition to using supplements this involves reducing the sugar in your diet since it is their food source. However, the Candida protocols are usually very simple. On the other hand, handling the issue of parasites is often as easy as simply taking the right supplement, finishing the bottle and being done with it. Healing intestinal permeability usually involves taking the right supplements as well.

After you first detox the intestines of parasites, yeast and constipation issues you can then focus on getting rid of intestinal permeability issues without worrying about the presence of invaders that might interfere with your efforts. That being said, let's look at some of the best protocols I've discovered over the years to handle each of these problems in turn.

## Eliminating Parasites

Parasite infections in the GI tract (and other areas of your body) are more common than you might think. They are a problem which particularly plagues international travelers, especially those who regularly visit underdeveloped countries. Eaters of exotic foods who stay at home can often find themselves with parasites as well.

Examples of parasites include pinworms, roundworms, tapeworms, whipworms, hookworms, blood flukes, Giardia (from drinking infected waters) and a variety of other critters that feed off you or your ingested nutrition. Bacterial parasites from travels can cause a wide variety of problems such as backpacker's diarrhea, the famous "Montezuma's Revenge" that happens to Mexico vacationers, or the travel diarrhea which frequently happens to visitors of exotic places such as India.

Many parasites can thrive in the body without showing any signs they are present. Others will cause you to immediately feel ill and suffer quite a few GI tract problems. There are all sorts of problems they can cause without you ever suspecting that parasites are the culprits. Some people, for instance, cannot gain weight or always feel empty after eating meals because parasites are feeding off their food, or they may be the cause of diarrhea that is just infrequent enough that you don't suspect their presence.

If you traveled abroad and then developed traveler's diarrhea during your visit or upon return, or presently have constant digestive issues and have tried countless methods to heal your gut to no avail, a good doctor will suspect a parasite issue. If you suffer from autoimmune conditions and various forms of mental distress, these are also red flags for the possibility of a parasite invasion.

The most common warning signs of a chronic parasitic infection are changes in the appearance or frequency of bowel movements (especially diarrhea or loose stools for two weeks), chronic exhaustion, sudden weight loss, itching around the anus, cramping and abdominal pain, unexplained constipation, skin irritations, grinding your teeth in your sleep, and aching muscles or joints.

How do you know for sure? You should ask your doctor to run a comprehensive stool test that visually looks for parasites or their eggs in your stool, and when appropriate you must check for their signs in your blood. Many tests use Polymerase Chain Reaction technology to discover the presence of parasite DNA or not. Once a physician tests you he/she will receive a full report and with those results can then prescribe a course of action. Always follow your doctor's orders in these matters.

The best way to get rid of parasites is through targeted prescription medications that your doctor specifies, especially since laboratory tests will often indicate which medications and/or natural supplements would be most successful in eliminating them. Some people don't really show any symptoms but because of their frequent travel lifestyle like to regularly do their own "parasite purges" at home by using powerful herbal formulas. Most of these natural parasite formulations will contain similar ingredients known to kill invaders such as black walnut hulls, sweet wormwood, cloves, bearberry, barberry, garlic, grapefruit, and tribulus.

There are many parasite detoxification herbal formulas on the market, but my favorite is PC123, which is available a BCN4life.com. Unlike other parasite cleanses it is a completely safe non-laxative formula that you can take on daily basis. The formula is the only one I know that is safe enough to be taken 365 days straight, and is excellent for correcting or *preventing* traveler's diarrhea. If you are going on a trip known to produce diarrhea you can take a bottle with you, use a dropper full twice per day, and prevent any problems of bacterial infections in the gut.

PC123 is an alcoholic tincture of special herbs that have been completely dissolved into liquid form. It is like a broad spectrum anti-microbial combination, but it does not seem to disturb good bacteria in the gut. The story goes that a pharmaceutical company came up with the base formula in 1988-89 that it sold for 10 years. They tested it against almost every gut pathogen they could find and it worked for everything including yeast, amoebas, protozoa and worms. It can and should be used for about a week before a Candida detox.

If you already have intestinal parasites, you need to consecutively take PC123 at least 60-90 days *non-stop* in order to kill any internal intestinal parasites that are there *and* their eggs, which might hatch weeks after you start an elimination program.

PC123 is gentler than most other anti-parasite formulas in terms of a die-off effect, and this is especially why I like it. Whether we are talking about amoebas, protozoa, yeast, or worms the PC123 formula seems to act on both the organisms and their larva without cracking their shells to produce a toxic response.

For me, the first step in an intestinal detox program is therefore to take two bottles of PC123 over the course of two months. Because I frequently travel overseas, this is what I personally do every now and then to help clean out anything that I may have picked up that might be trying to establish a beachhead inside.

## Eliminating Candida

Parasites are not the only invasive intestinal organisms that can negatively impact your health in a big way. Dr. William Cook made headlines years ago, capturing the attention of the medical community, after writing *The Yeast Connection* to alert everyone to the problems caused by the overgrowth of *Candida albicans* yeast in the GI tract. Skeptical that *Candida albicans* could cause major health issues, he put many of his chronically ill patients on a sugar-free diet (since sugar feeds yeast), gave them the anti-fungal drug Nystatin to kill off any yeast infections, and saw dramatic improvements in their health.

Cook's findings on the importance of reducing yeast overgrowth in your body were presented in *The Yeast Connection*, which sparked a revolution in our understanding of *Candida*-related GI issues. Since that time, countless articles on the dangers of yeast overgrowth have been published and the medical community now commonly recognizes its dangers.

Candida lives inside all of us, and Candida cells release up to 79 different types of toxic by-products in your blood as they go through their life cycle. Because they are continually reproducing and dying these toxins are constantly being released into your bloodstream to poison you. Those regularly released toxins can produce acne, eczema, fatigue, intestinal gas, stiff joints, brain fog and depression – all of which might be easily misdiagnosed or ignored by a physician. One of those toxins is acetaldehyde, which is transformed by your liver into alcohol and responsible for creating feelings of intoxication and brain fog.

Your liver has to detoxify all these poisons but can easily become overloaded if you develop a yeast overgrowth, in which case an excessive amount of toxins will daily pass through the liver untreated and produce symptoms such as constant fatigue, irritation, or foggy-headedness. Since these toxins must be processed by the liver, a good place to begin your detoxification program is in your bowel as we are doing. Decreasing the amount of these toxins will reduce the burden placed on your liver. Candida can actually cause your gut to become leaky, too, because it can burrow into the mucosa lining of your cell walls. The resulting inflammation will make the gut lining leaky and permeable. When you develop a leaky gut your problems start intensifying because large food molecules can then escape into your blood stream and the Candida can easily spread throughout your body.

Your chances of having yeast-connected health problems rise if you have taken a prolonged course of antibiotics, have intense sugar cravings and/or memory or concentration problems, often see a white coating on your tongue, suffer from chronic sinus and allergy issues, tend to feel "sick all over" or "feel sick all the time" without any specific causes, are frequently bothered by recurrent vaginal, prostate or urinary tract infections, experience recurrent hormonal imbalances, or are unusually sensitive to chemical odors such as perfumes or smoke. Antibiotics are the biggest concern, and many holistic doctors will put you on a course of probiotics during and after any course of antibiotics you take to kill infections.

Everyone has some degree of *Candida albicans* in their body, so the worry is yeast overgrowth rather than simply the presence of Candida. The best way to confirm whether you have a yeast overgrowth is to have a comprehensive stool analysis performed, which will usually also test which products would be the most effective in eliminating it. Many naturopaths and holistic physicians can authorize a "comprehensive stool analysis" for you using labs like Great Smokies Laboratory, Doctors Data, Great Plains Laboratory and so on.

Even if you use pharmaceutical anti-fungal agents like Diflucan or Nystatin to kill off Candida you cannot entirely get rid of yeast in your body. It has to be there because it is a natural part of your GI tract's biological terrain, which also includes a wide variety of bacteria and fungus. The problem arises only when there is yeast *overgrowth*, which typically happens when we consume too much sugar in our diets. Sugar is the fuel that feeds yeast and causes it to grow in the gut. If you eat too much sugar your yeast population might grow out of control.

Sugar has been identified as the main culprit behind countless diseases of the modern era. One hundred years ago we ate about four pounds per year of sugar whereas the average American now eats around 150-175 pounds of sugar annually. In addition to the fact we largely have sedentary lifestyles, this incredible amount of excessive sugar consumption accounts for our rising rates of obesity and diabetes.

The strategy for getting rid of yeast is fourfold: (1) starve the yeast with a low/no-sugar and no-yeast diet, (2) ingest supplements that kill it, (3) repopulate the gut with helpful probiotics, and (4) support the detoxification process by enhancing your liver function with supportive supplements during an anti-*Candida* campaign.

To free yourself of *Candida albicans* you need to cut down your consumption of sugar when undergoing any eradication protocol, otherwise you will be feeding the yeast while trying to kill it. You want to be on a sugar-free yeast-free diet.

In addition to the no sugar, no-yeast diet you need to give your intestines healthy probiotics such Pharmax HLC Multistrain, which is one of my favorites. Every few years the ranking of "best" probiotic companies seems to change among nutritionists and naturopaths, and Pharmax is the one I am using at the present. Many other probiotic products are also good such as Moss Nutrition's Probiotic Select and even Jarrow Formula's easily obtainable Jarro-Dophilus for those who don't have access to more proprietary brands. There are also probiotic strains used for specific purposes such as *Sacccharamyces boulardii* (Allergy Research) to help stop psoriasis. A holistic physician or skilled naturopath/nutritionist is the only one who can wisely advise you on a replacement probiotic.

The big nuisance about taking any pharmaceutical medications or natural supplements that kill Candida is the Herxheimer die-off reaction. As stated, there are 79 different toxins released by the metabolism and die-off of Candida, which is why people with a yeast overgrowth tend to feel so lousy. If you kill it too fast then a flood of those toxins will be released into your bloodstream en masse, and the response might be that you temporarily suffer from headaches, nausea, dizziness, joint or muscle pain, fever, chills or cold in your extremities, rashes or itchiness, skin breakouts, swollen glands, and recurring vaginal, prostate or sinus infections. This is called the Herxheimer reaction. It is unpleasant and typically lasts for 3-5 days.

Many natural products will kill yeast, but I favor those that produce less severe or *no* Herxheimer reactions at all as they do their work. A product that is particularly effective along these lines is Candisol (Candex is the consumer brand), which is one of the first products I would try for eliminating Candida. People who use Candisol will typically report very little of the Herxheimer die-off effect and often tell me that their mind seems to become more clear after three or four days of usage. That's a very good sign it is working.

If the Candisol/Candex doesn't seem like it is reducing the yeast to a manageable level then you might add "Physician's Strength Oregacillin" to the protocol. You would then be taking both Candisol and Physician's Strength Oregacillin at the same time to clear yourself of a stubborn Candida infection. Some of the other most effective herbs and substances for Candida include raw garlic, Venus Fly-trap extract, caprylic acid, Lomatium Dissectum (LDM-100) and wild crafted oregano (Oregamax), but you should start with Candisol and Oregacillin.

Another popular anti-Candida product is Candaclear Four by Pharmax. Composed of caprylic acid, allicin from garlic, cinnamon bark oil, and cinnamaldehydes, this product also eliminates the overgrowth of harmful organisms in the intestines. Also containing glutamine and n-acetyl glucosamine, it additionally helps to rebuild intestinal walls at the same time in order to reduce the risks of leaky gut syndrome. It also contains probiotics to help support microflora levels.

Years ago I would commonly use caprylic acid for yeast overgrowth problems, but for some reason it seemed to lose its effectiveness. Other nutritionists reported to me the same decline in results. However, a manufacturer who recently tested nearly one hundred brands finally found an exceptional one that seems to match its original effectiveness. This is now sold as the BCN Formulas Mojo Capyrlic acid that is available at BCN4Life.com.

One last note – anyone trying to eliminate Candida should

consider taking 400 mcg of high-selenium mustard greens (Phytosel) twice daily until the Candida symptoms are gone. High selenium mustard greens contain mostly l-selenocysteine. Selenium and cysteine are the best known precursors of glutathione, an intracellular cellular detoxifier, and glutathione and selenium together help your neutrophils control Candidiasis. No treatment for yeast overgrowth will last very long if you have depleted glutathione levels.

## Eliminating Constipation

As you know, constipation seems to be the most common issue of complaint when it comes to intestinal detoxification. Some researchers who have extensively studied aboriginal natives that still eat their traditional diet believe that a perfectly healthy body should have *at least* one bowel movement per meal. Chinese medicine, Indian Ayurveda and the Weston A. Price Nutritional Foundation agree, and commonly promote the idea that two or three daily bowel movements are healthier than just one per day. I agree, but many people don't have this many.

Conrad LeBeau, author the famous *Immune Restoration Handbook*, has reported that in his opinion a very healthy GI tract met the following requirements: the individual should have one or more bowel movements per day, they should be banana shaped, they should float rather than sink (sinking indicates the absence of friendly flora), they shouldn't stink or smell bad, they shouldn't be sitting on the toilet for more than two minutes maximum, and the individual pooping shouldn't have to use lots of toilet tissue to wipe themselves afterwards.

Most of us cannot possibly fulfill those healthy bowels requirements. In fact, many people cannot even come close so don't feel bad if that's you. Therefore physicians usually subscribe to the views of the ROME Multinational Consensus for defining constipation formulated in 2000, and updated in 2006, which states that constipation is having less than three bowel movements per week, straining more than 25% of the time, experiencing hard stools more than 25% of the time and incomplete evacuation more than 25% of the time.

Some doctors have an even simpler definition for constipation saying that if you are not passing stool (having a bowel movement) at least every third day then you are constipated. Of course, most people want to evacuate their bowels more frequently than this because it is uncomfortable, but for some people this is fine as long as they are not straining on the toilet and they completely evacuate their bowels at that time.

I personally like to hear that an individual has at least one bowel movement per day because most people feel better emptying with this regularity. Everyone feels better if they pass stool easily without straining, if it is soft rather than hard, and if they feel a sense of completion after elimination. If you are constipated, on the other hand, it often means that your bowel is packed with old fecal matter, some of which is reabsorbed through your intestinal walls into your blood vessels and recirculated.

What are the typical causes of constipation? It might arise from not eating a healthy diet, lacking sufficient fiber in your diet, not drinking enough liquids, not getting enough physical activity, having intestinal problems (rectal tumors or colon cancer, bowel obstruction, pelvic floor dysfunction, diverticulitis, Crohn's disease, etc.) or certain medical conditions (stroke, diabetes, scleroderma, multiple sclerosis, hypothyroidism, lupus). It can also be a side effect from taking certain medications.

For years, modern gastroenterology has taught that you could eliminate constipation by drinking more liquids and eating more fiber in your diet. Unfortunately, for many people this just doesn't work. Nevertheless, the fiber-rich foods recommended include beans, fresh fruits and vegetables, dried fruits, wheat bran, unrefined breakfast cereals, whole-grain bread and brown rice.

A popular fiber supplement used for constipation along these lines is psyllium seed, husk or powder form, which is the main ingredient of Metamucil. In fact, gastroenterologists love using psyllium seed powder for constipation. Psyllium powder is a great source of insoluble, non-digestible fiber that works by absorbing liquid and swelling in the intestines to create a bulkier, softer stool that is easy to pass. Once eaten, the mucilage swells to several times its size producing a bulky laxative that absorbs toxins and undesired elements in the colon. Psyllium powder has the benefit of acting as a non-harsh bulking agent that helps to scrape the plaque off intestinal walls without damaging them.

Whenever you swallow psyllium seed powder, husks or fiber you must always ingest a large amount of water because psyllium has a tendency to form large clumps that will stick to the sides of the small and large intestines when there isn't enough liquid. Therefore it can worsen the problem of constipation if you don't drink enough water when using it. The best practice is to take this type of product about an hour prior to eating.

Unfortunately, eating more fiber or even psyllium powder/husks doesn't work for everyone to end constipation or promote regular bowel movements. For some unlucky people this "orthodox" or "establishment" remedy even makes their constipation worse. Therefore, how might you approach the problem of constipation to achieve a "bowel detox" using a stronger routine that also detoxifies the intestines at the same time?

## Eliminating Mucoid Plaque

First, if at all possible you might consider a series of colonics or enemas to get rid of any impacted fecal waste on the walls of your colon. Colonics and enemas are therapies that use water inserted into the large intestine by way of the anal canal in order to wash your intestines. The water soaks and loosens hardened fecal debris that sloughs off the intestinal wall and is flushed out of the body when the water is evacuated.

As a healing therapy, enemas have been used for thousands of years to remove hardened fecal matter that would otherwise remain in the intestine and poison the body continuously while also contributing to constipation. Professionally administered colonics are superior to enemas as they enable water to reach and wash out the transverse colon, which is the last segment of the colon that home enemas may not reach.

This therapy, championed in the books of Edgar Cayce and Bernard Jenson (*Tissue Cleansing Through Bowel Management*) is something you do only at the beginning of a detox regime rather than all the time because it causes you to lose a lot of energy. Princess Diana was a proponent of colonics and attributed her beautiful complexion to frequently using this bowel cleansing technique that employs water to wash toxins and impacted fecal matter from the intestines.

I have personally seen skin conditions dramatically improve for people after they experienced just one colonic irrigation. When the fecal matter is removed from their intestines due to the water washing it away the beneficial results can be remarkable for your health. However, this procedure makes people feel like they lose energy and is only something I would do a few times at the beginning of a deep detox program. Colonics are not something I would use all the time with the frequency that Princess Diana employed.

Here is why colonics probably have such a striking result on the complexion. The capillaries in the mucosa lining of your rectum are not part of the body's hepatic portal system. Therefore when you are squeezing out stool through your rectum and anus, as it touches your intestinal walls (that have capillaries) toxins are normally reabsorbed into the body's blood supply, but in this case they bypass the liver and its detoxification functions.

The comfortable feelings from having passed stool not only arise because your bowels feel empty without the heaviness of obstruction, but also because after it is gone the poisons are no longer being reabsorbed from the circulatory system of the lower rectum and anus to then recirculate in the body.

If there is a lot of feces congestion in the large and small intestines due to constipation, then a significant amount of stool toxins will always be reabsorbed into your blood stream. Removing that constipation will reduce a source of recirculating toxins from your blood, and as a result mental feelings of heaviness or lethargy will disappear and your complexion will immediately brighten. People made fun of Princess Diana for using colon hydrotherapy on a frequent basis, but the fact is that she always looked radiant.

Our body is designed to expel stools as soon as possible after they arrive in the rectum, which is why curing constipation is important if you want to avoid the recirculation of fecal toxins. If the bowels are blocked or just slow, this gives a chance for the toxins to be reabsorbed and then shifted elsewhere in the body rather than expelled.

One of the major issues involved with constipation is mucoid plaque. Your body needs a certain degree of mucus as a lubricant for your stools and as a defense mechanism to stop pathogens and microbes from entering your body through the intestines. This is why your intestines are coated with mucosal cells that secrete fluids. Mucosal cells normally secrete mucus, but some foods such as dairy and soy products are especially mucus-forming.

As food particles move through your intestines, mixing together with the mucus they sometimes end up leaving a coating on intestinal walls rather than get excreted. As layers of mucus and food particles build up and dry out over time, the feces and mucus hardens to produce a tough, rubbery substance that forms clumps in the corners of the GI tract, coating its villi and walls.

This mucoid plaque prevents nutrients from being absorbed from the intestinal wall and can itself cause constipation. Over time, toxins and heavy metals become embedded into this mucoid plaque, which becomes a breeding ground for *Candida* and micro-organisms too. High fiber diets can help remove mucoid plaque from the intestinal walls and prevent its formation, but low fiber diets can exacerbate the problem.

While it is the liver's job to clear toxins from the blood, your liver depends on your kidneys and colon to efficiently eliminate toxins from the body. For the colon, this job is hampered if mucus and fecal matter start coating your intestinal wall, and autopsies typically show that around ten or more pounds of mucoid plaque usually coat a person's intestines. In excessive cases, the encrusted material can even amount to forty pounds or more! It makes sense to argue that some of it gets reabsorbed and recirculated into your bloodstream all the time.

How do you clear your intestinal tract of hardened feces and mucoid plaque, which contains toxins and harmful organisms and contributes to constipation? Normally a doctor would tell you to change your diet to add more fiber and liquids, or use Metamucil since it is largely made of psyllium seed husks that will scrape your intestinal walls. Here is where we can improve upon this basic advice.

It is often beneficial if you take psyllium seed powder together with liquid bentonite clay, which is a volcanic ash that absorbs toxins. The active ingredient within bentonite clay is montmorillonite, which can absorb many times its weight in bacteria and toxic materials found within the intestines. When hydrated with water, bentonite clay develops negatively charged particles while toxins and heavy metals have positive charges. This allows the bentonite clay to bind to the toxins and escort them from the body through the stool.

The best way to drink liquid bentonite as an intestinal detoxifier is on an empty stomach at least one hour before or after meals. The typical dosage is to mix one teaspoon to one tablespoon of bentonite clay with 8 ounces of water. Many people don't want to do any mixing themselves so they typically use Sonne's #7 Detoxificant, which already contains colloidal bentonite in liquid form.

When psyllium and bentonite clay are mixed together you can create a "P&B" shake to help clean the intestines. It will grind away at the intestinal walls, scraping the mucoid plaque off the walls without damaging them. This is more powerful a detoxifier than using just psyllium alone. When creating a P&B shake, liquid bentonite should be the first ingredient and then psyllium (that has already been mixed with water) should be added second. Once mixed you should drink immediately.

You can also add other ingredients to a P&B shake for cleaning the intestines, such as cayenne pepper to naturally stimulate the intestinal tract. Other fibers and absorbents that might also help to soften stools or loosen mucoid plaque include ground flaxseed, slippery elm bark, marshmallow root powder, acacia gum, and pectin powder.

The Ivy Bridges Formula is another drink you can put together yourself to help cleanse your bowels and flush encrusted and putrefied wastes from your colon. You should drink this formula every day for 30 days to cleanse and heal your colon. The formula is as follows:

½ cup apple juice
1 teaspoon psyllium powder
2 tablespoons liquid chlorophyll
2 tablespoons aloe vera juice
2 cascara sagrada capsules
1 glass of water

The recipe is to mix the apple juice, chlorophyll, aloe vera juice and psyllium powder together and drink immediately before the mixture thickens. This is followed by a full glass of water taken with two cascara sagrada capsules. It is best taken at night before sleeping so that you will have a full bowel elimination when you awaken in the morning

There are many products you can use to help cleanse and stimulate your intestinal tract, thus detoxifying your body of accumulated wastes. A variety of manufacturers have created simple to use intestinal cleaning kits that combine many of these ingredients together to help end constipation. The list of possibilities is by no means comprehensive, but includes:

Systemic Formulas "C-Colon"
Dr. Richard Schulze Intestinal #2
Jarrow Formulas Perfect Fiber
Blessed Herbs Colon Cleansing Kit
Dr. Natura's Colonix All Natural Intestinal Cleanser
Nature's Secret Ultimate Cleanse
Renew Life's Organic Bowel Cleanser

The Systemic Formulas "Colon" formula, consisting of pills, is the product I seem to employ most in my practice for clients with temporary constipation issues although sometimes I have used the herb turkey rhubarb.

Many individuals change their diet enough to avoid the technical definition of constipation, but even after increasing their fiber intake they might still only have one bowel movement in two or three days. To get rid of the constipation they often turn to laxatives, but an over-use of laxatives can lead to sluggish bowels and create dependency when the bowels begin to rely on this type of artificial stimulation.

Natural laxative supplements normally contain herbal components such as senna leaf, cascara segrada, or turkey rhubarb, and these are the ingredients that tend to make you dependent on the formulas, which also work less efficiently the longer you use them. Some ingredients, such as aloe, are much safer than senna compounds that particularly tend to produce dependency.

Yet another set of products that work together for constipation are a pair of Pure Body Institute formulations once again - "Indigest Free" and "Colon Booster," which have been relabeled as "Move More Fast." Indigest Free helps heal, repair and soothe the bowel (and is a mild parasite cleanse) while Colon Booster, containing fedegoso (a relative of senna), acts as an effective but non-addictive laxative. Used together, the two products often produce a powerful laxative response where other products fail, perhaps due to their unique blend of herbs which are not normally found in other formulations.

Triphala has also been used for thousands of years in Ayurvedic medicine as tonic for the lower GI tract to help with constipation issues. You take it in the morning or at night with warm lemon water. I don't have much experience with triphala, but this might be another avenue to pursue for constipation when these other formulas fail.

When people cannot do colonics or enemas, this is my short list of products I normally recommend to help people get their colons moving again to end constipation, cleanse the colon and intestines, and handle intestinal detoxification issues.

## Eliminating Intestinal Permeability

Intestinal permeability, or leaky gut syndrome, is the final factor to discuss that ties into the issues of intestinal detoxification and repair. This is a condition where holes form in our gut, allowing material to then regularly pass from inside the gastrointestinal tract out into the rest of the body. Because it is an enzyme cocktail, Vitalzym can sometimes intercept and destroy some of the particles that escape from the gut into the bloodstream, but you should focus on putting an end to the problem in the first place.

Candida overgrowth, intestinal parasites, bacteria, gluten, foods you are allergic to such as dairy, the onslaught of GMOs, chemicals, and stress are some of the many factors that can lead to intestinal permeability. It is often known to play a role in celiac disease, Crohn's disease, inflammatory bowel disease, irritable bowel syndrome, chronic fatigue, rheumatoid arthritis (inflammatory joint disease) and food allergies.

When you are detoxifying the intestines, killing off parasites and Candida, or simply helping to discharge mucoid plaque and impacted fecal matter build-up to eliminate constipation, you should address any leaky gut issues at the same time because of the damage that these other issues may have caused. Remember that detoxification also means supporting your organs of elimination, and addressing leaky gut is a matter of intestinal repair and support.

How do you know for sure that you have a leaky gut or not? An intestinal permeability test can confirm whether you have the condition. The test is easy to perform because it measures the presence of two sugars (lactulose and mannitol) in the urine via a urine sample collected six hours after ingesting them.

The next question is, how do you heal intestinal permeability if you have it? The answer is through intestinal repair supplements, whose major components should include pharmaceutical grade l-glutamine and n-acetyl-glucosamine. The other ingredients you will usually find in intestinal repair formulas include okra, mucin, gamma oryzanol, zinc l-carnosine, citrus pectin, aloe vera extract, slippery elm, marshmallow and others. As you might note, some of these ingredients regularly appear in constipation formulas.

I have used a number of products to help people suffering from intestinal permeability issues, and my short list of favorites include:

Genestine Permeability Complex
Pharmax Intestinal Purifier
Biogenesis Intestinal Repair Capsules
Moss Permeability Select
Designs for Health "GI-Revive"

These are all very powerful gut healers that may help a wide variety of common GI tract distress issues, and they generally tend to make people feel better after their usage. Sometimes they even help with constipation issues too.

A typical protocol is to first use one of these intestinal permeability supplements followed by a stomach supplement to help heal the upper gut. Hence, a client might go on 2 weeks of Genestine Permeability Complex followed by 2 months of AOR's Gastro Relief, which tends to help people with stomach issues. It's usually as simple as that.

In short, my typical intestinal detox selection includes 2 bottles of PC123 to eliminate parasites, Candisol (and possibly Physician's Strength Oregacillin) to eliminate Candida while on a no sugar diet, colonics or enemas to clean the colon if available, a mucoid plaque purge using a P&B shake for a number of days, and then an intestinal repair formula such as Biogenesis Intestinal Repair Capsules. This short list keeps things as simple as possible. You only need to use the protocols that are relevant to your situation.

# 4
# LIVER & GALLBLADDER CLEANSING

Now that we have handled colon and intestinal issues we come to the granddaddy of detoxification concerns, namely how to clean your liver. Your liver is your body's chief detoxification organ and poison control center. It is your liver's job is to detoxify (break down) toxic chemicals from both inside and outside of the body such as hormone residues, pollutants, medications, tobacco, alcohol, or chemical poisons. Most of those detoxified substances eventually make their way into your stool, which is why we handled colon detoxification first. I want to make sure that you first clear this major channel of elimination before we start dumping an increased amount of poisons into this channel.

Your liver also breaks down carbohydrates and proteins, cleanses your blood, and helps regulate your blood sugar. If we were to summarize its job we would say that it either tries to turn into fuel or excretes all the substances it comes into contact with.

Weighing about a pound, your liver is metabolically the most complex organ in your body, a virtual chemical laboratory that produces over 13,000 chemicals and 2,000 enzymes that assist the body's functions. It carries out over 500 vital life functions throughout the day. From these astounding numbers you can glean that its functioning is extremely important to the overall health of the body. If it isn't working well then you won't feel well or work well.

One of your liver's jobs is to create bile to help digest fats and the job of your gallbladder is to store this bile until it is needed.

When we eat foods that contain fats the bile is passed into the small intestine to aid digestion. Located on the undersurface of the liver, one of the gallbladder's greatest dangers is precipitating out stones due to the congestion of its contents. Once gallstones form in the gallbladder they will obstruct the flow of the bile needed by the intestines.

Surgeons commonly remove gallbladders in hospital operations to get rid of these gallstones when they cause discomfort, and after surgery patients need to take bile salt supplements (Allergy Research Ox Bile) for the rest of their lives to help digest fats. Few doctors tell patients this important fact, but doing so will greatly improve their digestion after surgery.

In terms of detoxification, your liver basically transforms toxic chemicals into water-soluble substances that can then be eliminated from the body. Although other organs also carry on detoxification work, your liver is the body's *master detoxification organ*. Since it is your chief detoxifier you want to do everything possible to support its health and well-being so that it is not overwhelmed by work and can optimally execute its many functions.

Since all of us are now being exposed to more chemical assaults than anytime previously in history, your liver is definitely being overworked from trying to perform its job. It should be supported and protected through herbal healing supplements and can use a periodic boost in its own cleansing. Most people have a liver that is overworked and congested with toxic wastes that it has been trying to eliminate from the body, but is too busy or weak to detoxify and discharge. It needs your help.

Unfortunately, hardly anyone bothers to help their liver do its job even though our livers are inundated with detoxification demands from ingesting too many harmful chemical residues, heavy metals, and inhalants from thousands of industrial and petrochemical products. Some of us drink alcohol or smoke tobacco, which make its work harder. All these demands make its job nearly impossible to perform optimally as in past ages unless it now gets some extra help. Luckily we can provide the liver with that needed assistance in the form of liver detoxification protocols and liver support supplements.

When it comes down to it there are just two major concerns with the liver we need to address: (1) liver and gallbladder cleansing and (2) liver support. There are individuals who need liver support in general because of a weak, dysfunctional or diseased liver, and there is the general need to cleanse the liver/gallbladder to assist their natural detoxification mechanisms (pathways and processes).

Chinese medicine, which normally treats the liver and gallbladder as a single unit, says that the way our liver communicates with us is by altering our emotions. Chinese medicine says that frequent anger and irritability are common signs of an unhealthy liver, weak liver or liver in trouble. Frequent mood swings or moodiness, emotional stress, irritability, depression, hot flashes, insomnia, fatigue, malaise, constipation, poor concentration and memory, brain fog, and skin problems are also signs of liver congestion and of your liver crying for help.

When your liver experiences toxic overload then it not only tends to cause emotional outbursts but can no longer play an effective role in detoxifying harmful substances and eliminating them from your body. Due to reduced liver efficiency, toxic substances will remain circulating in your blood negatively affecting every body cell, organ or tissue. According to the intensity of toxic exposure, liver damage may eventually manifest as hepatitis, liver cirrhosis, fatty liver, and other liver or biliary abnormalities.

Individuals with specific liver problems and chronic illness are likely to have liver detoxification issues, but the good news is that many types of health issues will improve or even disappear once the liver's toxic burdens decrease and it can catch up once again to its normal level of functioning. The liver has a remarkable ability to regenerate itself if its burdens are reduced and it is given the right supportive nutrients.

Another benefit to liver detoxification is that it is common for people to lose weight afterwards. Some of the many chemicals driving the obesity epidemic and blocking weight loss include plastics (BPA or phthalates causing endocrine problems), heavy metals, pesticides, mold and toxic beauty and body care products. These substances tend to turn on bad genes and turn off good genes in our bodies, and when your body can finally remove them because of detoxification you will often see dramatic weight loss.

## Interpreting Liver-Related Enzymes

To determine whether you have normal liver health and your

liver is functioning optimally you can check the levels of liver-related enzymes in your blood. However, you should use "optimal reference ranges" for blood markers that are developed from a population of very healthy people instead of from a general population containing sick individuals too.

Most blood test results list a "reference range" for blood markers but the rarely used "optimal reference ranges" are actually more accurate for doctors making medical diagnoses. They are much better indicators of health problems including sub-clinical conditions.

Such optimal ranges were first developed by Dr. Harry Eidinier[1] and are also featured in *Blood Chemistry and CBC Analysis* by Dick Weatherby and Scott Ferguson. These optimal reference ranges for blood markers can help people discover medical conditions that escape doctors who aren't using them.

Most doctors will tell you that an organ such as your liver or kidney might even be operating at a level 60-70% "below optimal" before its enzyme markers exceed the boundaries of normal blood reference ranges. In other words, doctors won't know the organs are in trouble until they have lost a lot of functionality and are in great jeopardy. If a physician uses these optimal ranges he or she will get have an early warning that something is going wrong if the blood markers exceed their ranges, thus giving you an earlier chance to intervene and fix things at the most treatable stage of a condition.

Hence, here is how you use these ranges. When your liver enzymes are abnormal it often indicates a dysfunctional, diseased, stressed or sluggish liver. When your enzymes exceed their optimal ranges on either the high or low end you need only read through the list of possible pathologies to get an idea of what may be wrong. Everyone should grab their latest blood chemistry lab report and look for abnormalities where the numbers are higher or lower (outside) than the optimal ranges and make note of the possible problems. When a large number of indications suggest the same problem, which matches with your other symptoms, then you can work with you doctor to start restoring things to normal.

These optimal blood chemistry ranges will be narrower than

---

[1] Dr. Harry Eidinier, *Balancing Body Chemistry with Nutrition Seminars*, "More than Just a Bunch of Numbers – Making Sense of Blood Chemistry Results" Quick Reference Guide, Second Revision, February 1998.

those found on ordinary blood test results so any range violations will usually tip people off to developing liver abnormalities earlier than if you used the ordinary ranges. If your liver enzymes are off, this may be a clue suggesting the need for liver support or liver detoxification. The optimal ranges for various liver-related enzymes (in American units) are as follows:

| | |
|---|---|
| SGOT (AST) | 10-30 |
| SGPT (ALT) | 10-30 |
| GGTP | 10-30 |
| LDH | 140-200 |
| Total Bilirubin | 0.1-1.2 (>2.6) |
| Direct Bilirubin | 0-0.2 (>0.8) |
| Indirect Bilirubin | 0.1-1.0 (>1.8) |
| Alk Phosphatase | 70-100 |
| Albumin | 4.0-5.0 |
| Platelet Count | 32-35 |

Here is the standard medical interpretation of reference range violations.

When GGTP exceeds the high end of the optimal range (>30) it is often indicative of liver cell damage, alcoholism, biliary obstruction, biliary stasis or insufficiency, mononucleosis, diabetes mellitus, epilepsy, acute or chronic pancreatitis, pancreatic insufficiency, or a dysfunction located outside the liver and inside the biliary tree. If GGTP levels are lower than the bottom of the optimal range (<10) then it could indicate a vitamin B6 deficiency or the need for magnesium (and sometimes vitamin A or K) supplementation.

When LDH is high (>200) it could indicate liver or gallbladder dysfunction, muscular dystrophy, acute hepatitis, mononucleosis, diabetes, hyperthyroidism, cardiovascular disease, vitamin B12 or folate anemia, tissue destruction or inflammation, or a viral infection. If LDH is lower than optimal (<140) this usually happens with reactive hypoglycemia, radiation toxicity and pancreatic dysfunction.

If the SGOT/AST measure is increased above the top of the optimal range (>30) then this could mean liver cell damage, liver dysfunction, dysfunction located outside the liver and biliary tree, hepatitis, alcoholism, or skeletal muscle damage such as excessive breakdown or turnover. It also happens from cardiac stress such as congestive heart failure, pulmonary embolism, an acute myocardial infarction or cardiovascular dysfunction. It could also be indicative of either infectious mononucleosis, the Epstein Barr virus or cytomegalovirus. If SGOT/AST is low (<10) then it could indicate alcoholism or a vitamin B6 deficiency.

When SGPT/ALT exceeds the high end of the optimal reference range (>30) this could be indicating hepatitis, liver dysfunction, liver cirrhosis, liver cell damage, a fatty liver, alcoholism, hepatitis, biliary tract obstruction, muscular dystrophy or excessive muscle breakdown or turnover. If SGPT/ALT is low (<10) it might indicate alcoholism, liver congestion, a vitamin B6 deficiency or a fatty liver.

When the total bilirubin measure exceeds the high end of the optimal range (>1.2) it could mean liver dysfunction, liver injury, jaundice, biliary tract obstruction or calculi (gallstones), biliary stasis, mononucleosis, hepatitis, oxidative stress, thymus dysfunction, RBC hemolysis, or Gilbert's syndrome. When the total bilirubin measure is lower than the optimal ranger (<.1) it could indicate spleen dysfunction or barbiturate/salicylate usage.

When the direct bilirubin measure is too high (>.2) it could be indicating biliary tract obstruction such as a tumor or biliary calculi.

When the indirect bilirubin measure is too high (>1.0) it might mean Gilbert's syndrome or RBC hemolysis.

When the Alkaline Phosphatase measure exceeds the upper border of the optimal range (>100) it could be the result of liver cell damage, liver cirrhosis, liver cancer, hepatitis, mononucleosis, biliary obstruction, Hodgkin's disease, bone growth or repair, congestive heart failure, leaky gut syndrome, adrenal cortex hyperfunction, herpes zoster, or metastatic bone carcinoma. When the Alkaline Phosphatase measure is decreased (<70) it could mean a zinc deficiency, celiac disease, hypochlorhydria, protein malnutrition, scurvy, osteolytic sarcoma, hypoparathyroidism, hypothyroidism, hypophosphatasia, nephritis, or folic acid anemia.

A sick liver also cannot have a high albumin level so albumin is a good marker for overall liver damage. When albumin is high (>5.0) it might mean dehydration, hypothyroidism, or lymphatic congestion but when albumin is low (<4.0) it could mean liver dysfunction, biliary cirrhosis, congestive heart failure, digestive inflammation, edema, pregnancy, oxidative stress, renal dysfunction, rheumatoid arthritis, hypochlorhydria, or the need for vitamin C.

The platelet count will also be low if there is full blown liver disease. For instance, if the liver gets damaged by hepatitis then there will be hepatic congestion and portal vein hypertension. This in turn leads to splenomegaly. As this occurs, platelets sequester leading to measurable thrombocytopenia. A low platelet count (<32) could also be indicative of anemias, leukemia, lupus, or rubella while it is often too high (>35) in cases of rheumatoid arthritis, polycythemia vera, low blood clotting function and anemias.

Many blood markers can indicate liver dysfunction other than the ones we have just focused on. For instance, the prothrombin time for blood clotting will also usually be elongated if the liver is damaged since the liver makes clotting factors. The point is that you can use a typical blood test to get an idea if your liver is running low in any way and needs some intervention from your behalf.

As a general rule, liver dysfunction will usually be indicated by high levels of LDH, SGPT/ALT, SGOT/ALT, bilirubin, direct bilirubin, serum iron, ferritin, and monocytes along with low levels of BUN, total protein, albumin, triglycerides and cholesterol. Liver cell damage will be indicated by high levels of total globulin, alkaline phosphatase, SGOT/AST, SGPT/ALT and GGTP.

The liver is an extremely resilient organ that can regenerate itself when given the chance, especially when provided the right protective and supportive supplements like alpha lipoic acid, silymarin (Milk Thistle extract) and especially BCM-95 curcumin (which is highly recommended). However, an even better step to helping a liver get well is often to lower its detoxification burden by cleansing the body of as many harmful substances as possible (including those within the liver), and then supporting it while it recovers. When your whole body is toxic your liver is working overtime and then it is time to detox your body and get a liver flush.

## A Basic Liver & Gallbladder Flush

Here is why people typically choose to do liver and gallbladder flushes. It is to empty the gallbladder of gallstones, help reduce the liver's toxic load and restore liver functioning to more optimal levels.

The liver's job includes cleansing our blood of impurities such as metabolic wastes, poisons and toxins. It neutralizes these wastes and even dumps some (such as bilirubin from destroyed red blood cells) into the gallbladder where they are stored for elimination. Mostly the gallbladder stores bile produced by the liver, but an excess of bilirubin, cholesterol or bile salts can build up inside it and thicken this material so that it turns into sludge and then clumps to form gallstones. Although rare, liver stones can also form in the liver when there is too much cholesterol in the body. Whenever any of these things happens your gallbladder and liver get backed up and congested, which is not exactly the best situation since the liver's job is to keep your blood and body clear of toxic poisons.

In more scientific terms we should say that mineral deposits, such as crystalized bile salts and gallstones, tend to accumulate over time in the gallbladder. A liver and gallbladder cleanse will expel any such materials that build up over time. In order to first soften any materials (stones) to make them easier to expel, you should for several days drink apple juice (which contains malic acid), take malic acid supplements, or ingest a healthy measure of phosphatidylcholine to soften the stones prior to a liver/gallbladder flush.

When it comes time for the liver/gallbladder cleanse, some people ingest Epsom salts to dilate the gallbladder tubes since they contain the mineral magnesium which acts as a muscle relaxant. The purpose is to prevent any gallstones from becoming trapped in the bile duct during a cleanse.

Physicians always warn that if your liver is too weak or you have large stones in your gallbladder then you do not want to do any flushes because the stones could get trapped in the narrow bile duct passageway, creating pain and possibly necessitating surgery. I have never actually heard of this happening to anyone, but everyone always cites this warning. In any case, you should work with a doctor or other qualified health practitioner who can evaluate your risks until you have completed at least two flushes. The method discussed here is one that holistic practitioners have used for years and is by far the quickest at getting the job done.

Adapted from instructions provided by Dr. David Williams, here are the standard directions for a liver and gallbladder flush:

1. For a Monday through Saturday noon, on an empty stomach drink as much organic apple juice or apple cider (which both contain malic acid) as your appetite allows in order to soften any

gall stones. 1-2 grams of malic acid per day is equivalent to a liter of apple juice. For the maximum amount of stone softening, you might add orthophosphoric acid drops (Phosfood Liquid available from Standard Process, or "Super Phos 30") to the apple juice for a total of 60 drops per day. The orthophosphoric acid works with the malic acid to dissolve and soften gallstones. Some people soften the stones by taking PhosChol (Nutrasal brand) in high doses several days before a flush as well. If you choose the orthophosphoric acid route, brush your teeth after drinking the apple juice and orthophosphoric acid mixture in order to prevent the acid from damaging your teeth.

2.  At noon on a Saturday, eat a normal but light lunch.

3.  Three hours after lunch, take 2 tablespoons of Epsom salts dissolved in a glass of cool water. Epson salts are available in most drug stores. You can use a shaker cup to dissolve the Epson salts, which taste better in cool rather than warm water. Epson salts, which contain magnesium, are an intestinal purge and also relax the muscles of the bile duct and gallbladder. As an intestinal purge the Epson salts induce diarrhea in order to flush out any gallstones once they have been purged. After drinking the Epson salts, rinse your mouth out with water.

4.  OPTIONAL: Four hours after lunch you might do a one pint (4 cups) coffee enema to stimulate your liver's release of bile and waste.

5.  Two hours later, take 2 tablespoons of Epson salts dissolved in cool water again. After drinking the Epson salts, rinse your mouth out with water.

6.  At bedtime, you can *quickly* drink either:

    a. ½ cup of unrefined olive oil mixed with ½ cup (a small glass) of orange juice, grapefruit juice or lemon juice. You can either stir them together, shake them together or mix them in a blender. Orange juice typically tastes best.

    b. ½ cup of warm unrefined olive oil blended with ½ cup of lemon juice.

    While inside your stomach and intestines, the olive oil in this mixture causes the liver ducts and gallbladder to contract and empty their contents into the duodenum, thus expelling their collection of gallstones and gall gravel. In other words the olive oil stimulates the gallbladder and liver to expel bile, which forces stones out of the gallbladder ducts. The citrus juice makes the oil easier to drink and speeds the transit of the olive oil through the stomach into the intestines, which helps to minimize nausea.

7. Rinse your teeth and then go to bed immediately. Lie on your right side in a fetal position with your right knee pulled up close to your chest for 20-30 minutes. Afterwards you can adopt your normal sleeping position, but it helps if you sleep on your right side (where your liver is located). If you feel like you want to have a bowel movement during the night then do what you must, but don't force anything. You also might feel nauseas due to the release of toxins from the liver and gallbladder.

8. The next morning, one hour before breakfast, take two tablespoons of Epson salts dissolved in cool water again. Later you can drink more water or orange juice as desired. Wait 2-3 hours before eating a light breakfast.

9. In the morning you might have diarrhea that will include soft, green pebble-like chunks that are the congealed olive oil. These are not gallstones or mineral deposits from the gallbladder, but actually the congealed olive oil.

10. OPTIONAL once again is to do another coffee enema (or hydrotherapy colon cleanse) after the liver/gallbladder cleanse has been completed to help remove any accumulated toxins/wastes in the colon.

This liver cleanse will purge the liver and gallbladder of a great many toxins. People usually repeat the liver flush several times every 2-4 weeks to help improve severe health problems. You can also drink the olive oil plus citrus juice mixture in the morning without all the other preparations, but just make sure that you are not too far away from a toilet on the day you do so because you never know when the urge to defecate will arise.

Truth be told, many people who perform a liver and gallbladder flush don't take any extensive precautions, especially if they have done one previously. They simply mix an 8 ounce cup of orange juice and lemon with olive oil in the proper proportion, drink it first thing in the morning, lie on their right side and then go about their business expecting that they will soon have to make a toilet visit to dump whatever is motivated to come out.

Such a simple liver detoxification protocol has been used by thousands of patients of Dr. Richard Shultz, who sells an excellent 5-day liver cleansing kit with accompanying liver detox herbs and tea. That's the kit I used for some of my first flushes because it makes everything easier. And one I still recommend today.

Another variant for stimulating the liver and gallbladder so that they discharge toxins - which is a technique long promoted by the medical establishment - is the coffee enema. The coffee enema is typically used by cancer patients (see my book *Super Cancer Fighters*) to help them deal with flushing out chemotherapy toxins.

## Coffee Enemas for Liver Detoxification

The purpose of the coffee enema is to use coffee to stimulate your liver to discharge its toxic wastes. With a coffee enema you absorb caffeine directly into your bloodstream through your intestines and when the caffeine makes contact with your liver it stimulates the liver causing it to discharge toxic materials into the intestines.

Coffee enemas are often portrayed as a bizarre aspect of holistic medicine but they come right out of the Merck Manual, which is the standard compilation of orthodox medical treatments. Therefore they are not some weird new detoxification therapy from left-field that was dreamed up by crazy holistic physicians and alternative medicine practitioners. They have actually been used by mainstream physicians in orthodox medicine for over fifty years to stimulate liver function and in turn, the processing and excretion of metabolic wastes from the body.

Coffee enemas are such a conventional medical treatment that the Merck Manual - the "Bible of the medical establishment" - advocated coffee enemas as a liver stimulant in all editions from the first printing in 1898 on through to 1977. They were routinely recommended in nursing texts too. The Gerson Cancer Institute has been recommending them for the past fifty years also.

Why their popularity? Because your liver is like a sponge that absorbs poisons if they are not detoxified and discharged, and coffee enemas cause the liver to expel those accumulated toxins, thus lowering its detoxification load. Coffee enemas have been proven to help patients eliminate toxic waste material from the body and improve their ability to deal with the burdens of detoxification.

The way a coffee enema works is that the coffee's caffeine, taken rectally as an enema, basically sets up a reflex that stimulates nerves in the lower bowel and various detoxification pathways in the liver. Dr. Peter Lechner reports that the palmitic acid in the coffee promotes the activity of the glutathione S-transferase enzyme, which detoxifies the liver. It increases the activity of this enzyme by 600-700%, which is extremely useful to the body's detoxification needs since the blood circulates through the liver roughly five times during the time that the coffee enema is being held inside.

A coffee enema is done by simmering coffee in distilled water, cooling it to room temperature, admitting it into your colon while lying on your back and then laying on your right side, retaining for 12-15 minutes. The exact administration instructions are as follows:

- Add 3 tablespoons of fresh ground organic coffee to 1 quart of purified/distilled water. Do not use pre-ground coffee beans but grind the beans fresh. You should always use organic coffee that is caffeinated, never decaffeinated or the cheap instant coffee form the supermarket. Boil for 3-5 minutes to drive off the oils and then cover it with a lid and simmer for 15 minutes.
- Strain the coffee by passing it through gauze or an organic (non-bleached) coffee filter to remove large particles, and then allow it to cool to a comfortable body temperature. Never use it steaming hot. Put this in an enema bag that you hang elevated above you, whether you are standing, lying down and so on.
- Next lie down, lubricate the nozzle and insert it several inches into the rectum. Allow the coffee to drain very slowly into your intestines; use the clamp to adjust the speed of the flow. Relax and breath slowly while it goes into your intestine.
- Try to take in the whole bag and retain the coffee for around 15 minutes. If you feel spasms or unpleasant symptoms, close the clamp or lower the bag to the floor to stop the flow. Wait for half a minute and then try again. Sometimes gently massaging your belly will help you absorb more coffee.
- People who are ill may do this two or three times daily, or as needed. If you feel any immediate discomfort or experience a fever or headache, nausea, intestinal spasms and drowsiness,

it generally indicates the successful flushing of toxins from your liver. You should increase the frequency of enemas if this happens because these symptoms indicate that you need more. You might try adding an extra enema at night before sleeping.

- After the last enema, you should inject about 50 ml of cold-pressed, organic sunflower seed oil, flaxseed oil or similar into your rectum to line your intestines and protect their mucus membranes.

After you do your first coffee enema and attain some familiarity with the process, it becomes very easy to repeat it on a frequent basis. Cancer patients are told to do one every day. Its effectiveness in stimulating the liver to discharge wastes and improve its detoxification abilities is the reason why it has been adopted as a standard practice by numerous cancer clinics all over the world. As detailed in *Super Cancer Fighters*, this is an adjunctive at home cancer remedy that can help people deal with the side effects of conventional cancer therapies such as chemotherapy.

## Morning Liver Flush Drink

A final type of liver cleanse and support is a lemon/olive oil drink that you can drink on a daily basis. First brought to my attention by the *Immune Restoration Handbook*, this drink was designed to produce significant improvements in the detoxification of the liver and lymphatic system. This liver flush drink also helps to decrease the size of swollen lymph nodes, which are a sign of liver congestion.

Dr. Philip Princetta reported that when the liver is flushed out with the drink, the lymph fluid moves into the liver to be processed and its poisons are then eliminated from the body. It has an incredible track record in helping cancer, AIDS, and chronic fatigue immune dysfunction patients.

It is sometimes called the Whole Lemon drink because to make it you cut up one medium lemon into quarters and place them in a blender.

Next, you must add one cup of orange juice, red grape juice or other fruit juice. Then add one tablespoon of cold pressed extra virgin olive oil.

Next, optionally add one half-inch of raw ginger root which will help you digest the olive oil. You might also add one garlic clove, but this is optional too.

Blend at high speed for 1-2 minutes, pour the mixture through a strainer to separate the juice from pulp, discard the pulp and then drink all at once first thing in the morning.

## Liver Detoxification Herbs

Some people don't want to do any of these flushes and just prefer the route of taking liver detoxification herbal supplements. When you want to detoxify your liver you must remember that there are two approaches: (1) coarse liver dredging (2) and fine dredging of the liver.

Coarse dredging includes things like the liver/gallbladder cleanse or coffee enema that causes a rapid discharge of many liver toxins. Fine dredging includes "light" detoxification protocols such as the use of Pekana's apo-Hepat spagyric drops or the Herbalist and Alchemist brand Milk Thistle Extract.

A moderate level of dredging and support would be to use vitamins or herbs to slowly detoxify the liver such as found within Designs For Health LV-GB Complex, Pure Body Institute Liver Balance Plus, or Thorne's Liver Cleanse. Products like Rowachol, which helps dissolve gallstones in the biliary tract by increasing the solubility of the cholesterol in the bile, also fall into this category.

Even the Edgar Cayce practice of a castor oil pack held on top of the liver can be considered a mild form of liver detoxification therapy. Castor oil packs are a miracle remedy for shrinking cysts and tumors and dissolving scar tissue. You can find out more about the incredible usefulness of castor oil packs in Dr. William McGarey's *Edgar Cayce and the Palma Christi.*

## Liver Support

Lastly we come to the topic of herbal and vitamin liver support, and for this we must definitely turn to traditional herbal formulas that also contain some nutritional ingredients. Typically you should use herbs and supplements to support your liver for one or two months *before* you undertake any serious detoxification protocol. The liver will even start to cleanse and heal itself on its own if you do this to help protect/support it and take the detoxification load off for awhile.

When it comes right down to it, most liver products generally are built on a foundation of NAC and alpha lipoic acid with other minor ingredients thrown in to help normalize liver function. Therefore most liver support formulas will contain ingredients from the following list: alpha lipoic acid, N-acetyl-cysteine (NAC), glutathione, milk thistle extract (silymarin), bupleurium, rehmannia root, berberine, dandelion root, beet root, barberry, artichoke, burdock, turmeric, SAMe, calcium d-glucarate, methionine, choline, reishi mushrooms, phosphatidylcholine and so on.

Most of these ingredients serves a special liver *protectant* function rather than cleansing or healing function. All sorts of herbs and substances serve as liver protectants so that it can devote time to self-healing, but they are not necessary rejuvenators or cleansers. For instance, silymarin protects the liver from damage by coating liver cell walls and preventing toxins from entering but is not really a detoxifier. Phosphatidylcholine (I like the Nutrasal PPC brand – see phoschol.com) is another helpful natural substance that acts as a liver protectant against alcohol, pharmaceutical drugs, pollutants, viruses and other toxic influences. Alpha lipoic acid is a little different because it is also a repair assistant that can stimulate liver regeneration.

Liver disease pioneer Dr. Burt Berkson, author of *The Lipoic Acid Breakthrough*, discovered the extreme usefulness of alpha lipoic acid for liver detoxification and regeneration when he saved several patients from mushroom poisoning that was destroying their livers. Over the years he has developed various liver healing and support protocols that usually involve the trio of alpha lipoic acid, milk thistle (silymarin), and selenium. The selenium I always use is the Phytosel brand made from hydroponically grown mustard greens that absorb a high content of selenium.

You can find combinations of these ingredients in a variety of liver support/cleanse formulas, and truth be told it is difficult to say which is best so I rotate them when doing a liver detox on myself. New ones are always being invented and popular ones currently include Lipotropic Complex (Integrative Therapeutics), Liver Cleanse (Thorne), LV-GB Complex (Designs for Health), Liver GI Detox (Pure Encapsulations), Liver Detox (Protocol for Life Balance), Liver

Support (Vital Nutrients), Liver-Balance Plus, Himalayan "Liv52" and Nutrasal Liverflo. In particular, Nutrasal Liverflo contains four individual compounds (PPC, SAMe, silymarin and glycyrrhizin) that stimulate the detoxification *and* regenerative powers of the liver.

As gentle support and drainage products for the liver I like to use apo-Hepat and Apex's TerrainMax Liver Terrain formula.

One of the substances that greatly helps with liver detoxification is glutathione, but it is not something you should use without first having cleansed the liver for awhile. Glutathione is a super strong antioxidant that is the body's main cellular detoxifier. One of its jobs is to bond with toxins to form a water-soluble complex that is excreted through the liver, and during detoxification your body never seems to have enough of it.

A *deep* liver detox program should actually be accompanied by glutathione supplementation due to the assistance it can render, but oral supplementation does a poor job of boosting glutathione levels within the body. Doctors will tell you that you can only boost your glutathione levels through an IV, but this isn't exactly true. The oral supplements that actually work best are liposomal glutathione products so when your liver is really in trouble these are what you should use. Popular glutathione supplements that will help with liver detoxification include:

Valimenta Liposomal Glutathione
ReadiSorb Liposomal Glutathione
Pure Encapsulations Liposomal Glutathione
EuroMedica Clinical Glutathione

The less glutathione available to your cells, the longer any cellular detoxification program will take, which is why glutathione supplementation is suggested during deep cellular liver detoxes. If you proceed at an aggressive detoxification pace regardless of glutathione levels, sooner or later the body will run very low, opening up the possibility of liver stress on account of the lack of the protection offered by glutathione.

In this chemical age your liver's detoxification systems are easily overloaded. Your liver is being overworked in its role as the body's main organ of detoxification. When it isn't functioning at its best it cannot take care of the body properly. Hence you should help it periodically by doing a detox.

When I personally want to do a liver detox I make it very simple. I perform a liver and gallbladder flush using the Dr. Richard Schulze kit, and then I also take some form of liver detoxification tablets from the list previously mentioned. If I want to undertake a very long or deep liver or kidney detoxification program then I remind myself that I'm not in a rush. I typically kick it off using two or more months of support formulas such as these so that I don't overload the organs when I finally get down to the real dirty work of heavy detoxification. That's when I do a flush and afterwards call on liposomal glutathione and other stronger detox products.

It is almost impossible to say which of these liver support formulas is best so I typically rotate the ones I take each time I do a liver flush and liver detox program. The key, however, is to start with a simple liver and gallbladder cleanse whether using olive oil or he coffee enema.

# 5
# KIDNEY AND BLADDER DETOXIFICATION

The last part of our "master detoxification trio" are the kidneys. The kidneys are two bean-shaped organs, one on each side of the spine located high in the abdominal cavity, which play a major role in cleansing your blood of harmful elements. Among other functions (such as regulating the body's pH and electrolyte balance), they continuously regulate your blood's chemical composition by filtering it to remove waste products. The wastes are then excreted into the urine.

We would soon be poisoned by our own wastes if the kidneys stopped filtering our blood. The wastes excreted by the kidneys into your urine include, among other things, urea from breaking down proteins and uric acid from nucleic acid metabolism. If you don't drink enough water, inside the kidney's nephron tubules these toxic solutes can become concentrated like sludge. This can then lead to kidney stones, infections and other sorts of damage that will weaken your kidneys and produce various sorts of renal dysfunction. However, your kidneys can lose 80% of their functional ability before symptoms appear, which is why kidney disease is usually at an advanced stage before its presence is detected.

At any moment in time you can find about 20-25% of your body's total blood supply being filtered in your kidneys. The two kidneys cleanse the entire blood supply of your body about 300 times per day, and the amount of work they perform is based upon the amount of dissolved substances and urea they must remove from the blood.

Dependent upon fluid flow to do their job, drinking too much or too little water or other liquids can overstress the kidneys. Some common signs of kidney stress include bags under the eyes or pain on one or both sides of the spine where they are located. When people suffer from lower back pain or low sex drive, Chinese medicine says that weak kidneys are the cause with the common remedy being kidney detoxification and support to strengthen them.

Not only must we drink enough liquids to avoid kidney problems but we should take regular steps to help detoxify them in order to insure their optimal functioning, reduce their burden, prevent problems like kidney stones from building up, and prevent them from weakening due to overwork or chemical assault. When kidneys are considered weak or damaged most holistic health practitioners will take detoxification and support steps to help restore kidney health.

Modern western doctors usually cannot make any conclusions about someone's kidney health unless they perform various lab tests to test their functioning, such as urine exams or blood chemistries. As taught, blood chemistry reports should use "optimal ranges" as the reference ranges for blood markers to determine your true state of kidney health.

The *optimal* reference ranges for measuring your kidney health (and thus tipping you off to the interventional need for detoxification or support) are as follows:

| | |
|---|---|
| BUN | 10-16 |
| BUN/Creatinine | 10-16 |
| Creatinine | 0.8-1.1 |
| Uric Acid | 3.5-5.9 male; 3.0-5.5 female |

When BUN levels are higher than the upper bounds of the optimal range (>16) this can be indicative of renal disease, renal insufficiency and other types of renal dysfunction. It is also indicative of dehydration, hypochlorhydria, excessive protein diets, adrenal hyperfunction, dysbiosis, edema, or anterior pituitary dysfunction. Low BUN levels (<10) can be indicative of low protein diets, malabsorption issues, pancreatic insufficiency or liver dysfunction.

When creatinine is high (>1.1) this is usually found in conditions of severe nephritis, prostate hypertrophy, urinary tract congestion, renal disease, starvation, gout, renal insufficiency or uterine hypertrophy. When creatinine levels are low (<.8) it is often indicative of muscle atrophy, pregnancy or bone growth.

When the Bun/Creatinine ratio is excessively high (>16) it is sometimes indicative of kidney disease, urinary tract obstruction, prostatic hypertrophy, internal bleeding, burns, dehydration, fever, and when low (<10) it sometimes identifies either a low protein diet or posterior pituitary dysfunction.

When uric acid levels are high (>5.5 for females or >5.9 for men) this is often found in conditions of acute and chronic nephritis, mercury or lead poisoning, hypertension, gout, atherosclerosis, rheumatoid arthritis, oxidative stress, renal insufficiency, renal disease, circulatory disorders, leukemia, malignant tumors, and leaky gut syndrome. Uric acid levels too low (<3.0 for females or <3.5 for men) are typical when individuals suffer from molybdenum deficiency, B12/folate deficiency anemia, or copper deficiency.

As a general rule, renal disease is usually accompanied by high levels of uric acid, phosphorus, LDH, SGOT/AST, BUN, creatinine, the BUN/Creatinine ratio and magnesium. Renal insufficiency is usually accompanied by high levels of BUN and phosphorus and possibly higher levels of uric acid and creatinine (that may remain normal). By examining your blood marker ranges you will have a good idea as to whether you should be placing a special health emphasis on your kidneys and whether they need assistance with detoxification or support.

In many cases individuals suffering from kidney disease have been exposed to toxic heavy metals and show arsenic in their hair. Heavy metals such as cadmium, nickel, chromium and lead, which are used in fertilizers in some countries, are often the culprit. In a later chapter we will cover the topic of heavy metal detoxification protocols but you should first understand simple kidney detoxification regimes.

## Kidney Cleansing

As with the liver, there are two major ways you can boost kidney health, which is through (1) kidney cleansing and (2) kidney support. Kidney protocols in general are usually a lot less complicated then those involved with detoxifying and helping to regenerate your liver.

To help detox your kidneys you should drink plenty of water every day. Many people squeeze a half lemon in a glass of water and drink this every morning as a simple ongoing kidney detoxification routine.

You can also drink special herbal teas made specifically for kidney and bladder detox efforts. They usually contain herbs like uva-ursi, juniper berry, hydrangea root, gravel root, parsley, horsetail, cornsilk, goldenrod, lobelia, or marshmallow root that help support or cleanse the kidney and bladder. I once heard of an individual curing their bladder cancer by drinking MesoPlatinum colloidal platinum from PurestColloids.com, and you can find a variety of cancer helps in my book *Super Cancer Fighters*.

Herbalist Dr. Richard Schulze produces his own kidney-bladder flush tea ("K-B Tea") containing some of the major kidney cleansing and support ingredients, and I continue to use it as a standard because I have seen it produce incredible healing results. I always use this tea in my detoxification programs and personally take it at least once a year as a kidney cleanse. The other special herbal tea I drink once or twice a year is Essiac Ojibwa tea.

Many supplement manufacturers offer powerful formulas to help with kidney cleansing and detoxification. The ones I use most often include:

Dr. Schulze K-B (Kidney-Bladder) Tea

Pekana's Renelix, a sphageric formula that is one of the best kidney drainage formulas in existence

Rowatinex, a natural formula used to dissolve and prevent the formation of kidney stones

Together with the herb chanca piedra (AOR brand or Raintree Nutrition) I also sometimes use pharmaceutical grade free form glycine (Freeda brand) at 5 grams per day in divided doses (1/2 teaspoon in the morning and ½ teaspoon at night) to protect and clean the kidneys and liver. Glycine supports healthy kidney and liver function by supporting the detoxification of certain chemicals. It combines with many toxic substances and converts them into less harmful forms to be excreted from the body. You can put the glycine in water or juice but should not take it with a protein meal.

## Kidney Support Formulas

When the kidneys are weak they usually need nutritional support for their tissue integrity or for normalizing their functional processes. Herbs and gentle homeopathic formulas are usually the safest ways to support your kidneys and urinary tract.

Chinese medicine has a number of formulas that support and boost kidney function too, but you need a skilled TCM practitioner to prescribe the right one for you. Without that guidance, it is hard to pick the right Chinese formula.

Typically I restrict myself to selecting from the following remedies to support weak, diseased or dysfunctional kidneys:

Systemic Formulas "K-Kidney" or "Ks-Kidney S"
Balanceuticals NephroEase (great for dialysis support)
Dr. Schulze K-B Kidney-Bladder Tea
Apex Energetics "Kidney Terrain (T12)"
Pekana Renelix

In Chinese medicine the kidneys are considered the foundation of good health and vitality, are related to hearing, and as the liver is related to the emotion of anger the kidneys are related to the emotion of fear that depletes their energy. The kidneys are also related to the strength of sexual function. If any of these areas are weak or dysfunctional then it often denotes the need for kidney support, especially if the relevant kidney enzymes also indicate a problem.

## Eliminating Kidney Stones

Painful kidney stones are another problem that is a "detoxification" concern. About 20% of men and 10% of women are expected to suffer from a kidney stone during their lifetime, which is twice the amount of thirty years ago. Isn't there something we can do about this?

The herbs chanca piedra, hydrangea root and gravel root are commonly used to break up and dissolve kidney stones, as does the natural formula Rowatinex. Melon seed tea and celery seed tea are also said to help dissolve kidney stones too. Out of all these choices, chanca piedra is the herb I suggest you concentrate on as it will help detox both the kidneys and liver. Two of the best brands are AOR or Raintree Nutrition.

When I want to go on a *deep* kidney detox I always do some preparatory herbal work first. I first use chanca piedra to break up any kidney (and gallbladder) stones that might be forming and start taking the herb one or two weeks before the flush along with glycine, which together will both protect and cleanse the kidneys and liver. Planetary Formulas Stone Free also helps to break up kidney and gallbladder stones.

Only afterwards do I use a package of Dr. Schulze's Kidney-Bladder tea for my kidney-bladder detoxification flush, along with a half lemon in a glass of water every morning. The protocol is therefore to first do some work to break up stone and then do further work to help flush them out with the tea.

One bit of additional information in regards to kidney stones. Some doctors may warn that large doses of vitamin C will cause kidney stones when in fact vitamin C does *not* cause kidney stones! Vitamin C increases urine flow, lowers urine pH, and prevents calcium from binding with urinary oxalate. All of these characteristics prevent kidney stones from forming and the kidney stone/vitamin C warning is a myth.

## Eliminating Kidney, Bladder and Urinary Tract Infections

A final note should be made about how to help heal urinary tract infections (UTI), which is the second most popular type of infection in the body. This is a common kidney-bladder problem that can usually be helped holistically when antibiotics fail and nothing else seems to work.

While normally treated with antibiotics, Dr. Jonathan Wright (a pioneer in nutritional-based medicine) says that the initial treatment of choice for most urinary tract infections should be the simple sugar D-mannose. Using D-mannose (powder in water or capsules) can actually knock out such infections where antibiotics have failed.

When we take a large quantity of D-mannose almost all of it spills into the urine through our kidneys, literally "coating" any E. coli bacteria present, which are the bacteria that cause 90% of UTIs, so that they can no longer "stick" to the inside walls of the bladder and urinary tract. The E. coli are then literally rinsed away during normal urination thus stopping infections in their tracts!

Dr. Jonathan Wright was one of the first physicians to start using D-mannose to treat UTI patients. For the treatment of UTIs he uses 1 teaspoon (abut 2 grams) for adults or ½ to 1 teaspoon for children, dissolved in a glass of water and repeated every two to three hours. Patients are told to continue with this for two to three days after symptoms have disappeared. D-mannose can be combined with the K-B tea so that this team becomes a double whammy to stop chronic kidney, bladder or urinary tract infections.

# 6
# ARTERIAL CLEANSING

Cardiovascular disease, and in particular heart attacks and strokes, is the #1 cause of death in America. It is typically caused by the build-up of cholesterol on inner arterial walls which become clogged with plaque. The problem starts on the inner lining of the arterial wall which consists of a layer of endothelial cells that prevent toxic substances from penetrating the smooth muscle of the blood vessel. As we age a host of factors can damage those endothelial cells such as circulatory poisons, free radicals, sugar, smoke and infections.

When toxins penetrate the layer of endothelial cells this produces an inflammatory response that causes cholesterol deposits to appear in order to repair the damage. Over time the cholesterol plaques get larger and then they calcify causing arterial disease. Sometimes the plaques rupture, which can produce deadly blood clots or stroke.

If we are talking about arterial detoxification we have to address how you can cleanse your blood vessels of this type of build-up. A detoxification strategy for arterial health means any natural methods that restore arterial integrity by reducing plaques, calcification and blood clots. Arterial cleansing basically means that you want to unclog (clean out) your blood vessels using any natural means available. Luckily such methods are available.

Many factors directly contribute to the dysfunction of the endothelial cells in blood vessels, but luckily you can get a tip-off to the risk of vascular disease through standard blood tests. After examining a standard blood test you can see what risk factors are out of bounds and can then develop a targeted intervention strategy to address the factors that are falling outside of their optimal ranges. The "optimal" Harry Eidinier ranges for several important blood markers connected with heart health are as follows:

| | |
|---|---|
| LDL | <120 |
| HDL | >55 |
| Total Cholesterol | 150-220 |
| Trigylcerides | 70-110 |
| Glucose | 80-100 |

The way to interpret these factors is as follows.

When LDL levels exceed the high of the optimal range (>120) this could be a sign of atherosclerosis, fatty liver, hyperlipidemia, oxidative stress or a diet too rich in carbohydrates. LDL levels are important because when LDL penetrates the endothelial wall it forms the core of plaque deposits and triggers an inflammatory response that accelerates vascular disease.

When HDL levels are much too high this could be the result of an autoimmune process. When HDL levels are too low (<55) this could be indicative of atherosclerosis, diabetes, a fatty liver, heavy metals, hyperlipidemia, oxidative stress, hyperthyroidism, obesity or too little exercise.

High levels of total cholesterol (>220) are typically found in cases of atherosclerosis, cardiovascular disease, celiac disease, biliary duct obstruction, liver disease, lipemia, leukemia, hypothyroidism, adrenal cortical dysfunction, insulin resistance, diabetes mellitus, fatty liver, multiple sclerosis, hyperliproteinemia, nephrosis, jaundice, and renal dysfunction. When total cholesterol drops below the lower bound of the optimal range (<150) it is sometimes indicative of thyroid hyperfunction, adrenal hyperfunction, hepatitis, shingles, uremia, polycythemia, low libido, epilepsy, endocrine dysfunction, autoimmune processes, oxidative stress, heavy metals, liver or gallbladder dysfunction, or malnutrition.

When triglyceride levels are higher than the top of the optimal range (>110) this is often the result of atherosclerosis, cardiovascular disease, insulin resistance, diets high in carbohydrates, thyroid hypofunction, liver congestion or a fatty liver, poor fat metabolism, early stage diabetes, hyperlipidemia, hyperlipoproteinemia, primary hypothyroidism, adrenal cortical dysfunction, or alcoholism. When triglyceride levels are below the low end (<70) this usually shows up as the result of thyroid hyperfunction, adrenal hyperfunction, vegetarian diets, autoimmune processes, free radical pathology or liver dysfunction.

If glucose levels are too high (>100) it could be indicative of early stage diabetes, a fatty liver or liver congestion, asthma, cerebral lesions, coronary thrombosis, diabetes mellitus, nephritis, a potassium deficiency, uremia, urinary obstruction, insulin resistance, cortisol resistance or a thiamine deficiency. Elevated glucose levels typically accelerate the microvascular damage of atherosclerosis and endothelial dysfunction. When glucose is below the lower bound of the optimal range (<80) it could be a sign of hypoglycemia, mumps, Addison's disease, starvation, pancreatic adenoma, hepatic insufficiency, adrenal hypofunction or hyperinsulinism.

In general atherosclerosis is usually accompanied by low levels of HDL and high levels of triglycerides, LDL, uric acid, platelets, and cholesterol (which possibly may show normal levels).

These aren't the only heart health indicators that you should monitor for early signs of cardiovascular disease. There are a variety of other blood markers that will indicate the need for a cardiovascular nutritional intervention strategy such as levels of fibrinogen, Lp(a), homocysteine and C-reactive protein (CRP).

Now that we have the blood markers for the important indicators directly related to cardiovascular health, however, if we want to clean our blood vessels of excess cholesterol plaque, calcium and blood clots, where should we start?

Each of these problems can be handled via natural means. Blood clots in the arteries and veins can be reduced using the supplement nattokinase, the calcination of plaques can be reduced via EDTA chelation therapies, and a variety of vitamin supplements (the "orthomolecular approach") can be used to reduce atherosclerotic plaque in general.

## Eliminating Blood Clots

To clean out your arteries and veins one of the easiest ways to start is by using nattokinase, an over-the-counter enzyme supplement that can prevent and dissolve blood clots while boosting other clot-dissolving agents.

Derived from the fermentation of natto beans, nattokinase (Allergy Research/Nutricology brand) is a natural oral clot busting product that dissolves blood clots better than pharmaceutical drugs. It was discovered over twenty years ago by Japanese researcher Dr. Hiroyuki Sumi when he was searching for a natural agent that could successfully dissolve blood clots associated with heart attacks and stroke. Although a natural supplement, it is commonly recommended by holistic physicians for patients with a medical history of stroke or blood clots, coronary artery disease, dementia, or elevated Lp(a) - a lipid that leads to hypercoagulability (sticky blood). Dr. Joseph Mercola reports that it even builds your bones better than calcium!

A variety of animal and human trials have definitively shown that nattokinase thins the blood and internally dissolves the fibrin and plasmin of blood clots. In fact, Japanese researchers have shown that 100 grams of natto exhibit the same fibrinolytic (clot dissolving) activity as a therapeutic dose of urokinase, which is a man-made product used to dissolve blood clots in the lungs. However, nattokinase stays active in the body for 8-12 hours while urokinase is active for less than an hour, and nattokinase costs far, far less. Nattokinase has similar blood thinning effects to aspirin, but it improves blood flow in the body without adverse side effects such as bleeding or gastric ulcers.

People take nattokinase for a variety of health conditions including high blood pressure, stroke, chest pain, hemorrhoids, heart disease and poor circulation. Every year I personally use it as an internal blood clot cleaner for preventive purposes. Before taking this nutritional supplement people should check with their doctors, who will most likely tell you to avoid it if you are taking a blood thinner such as Coumadin (warfarin) since both products will thin the blood to reduce blood pressure.

Nattokinase is an enzyme that fits well with Vitalzym since the Vitalzym will eat away at all the micro-fibrin plugs clogging up the micro-circulation of your blood vessels. Given enough time Vitalzym will also eat away at any scar tissue including even those within the filtering fingers within your kidneys (glomerulosclerosis). After several weeks of usage it is common for people to feel greater warmth in their hands and legs and experience lower blood pressure because of better blood flow. This is why both nattokinase and Vitalzym are a great combination that not only reduces blood clots within the blood vessels but help reduce high blood pressure.

## Eliminating Atherosclerosis

Our second cardiovascular condition to worry about is the buildup of cholesterol plaque on arterial walls. Many people think of the narrowing of arteries due to plaque buildup – a condition called "atherosclerosis" that is the basis behind many cardiovascular diseases - through the analogy of plumbing. They typically think of arteries as stiff pipes that gradually become clogged with blood clots, excess cholesterol and mineral deposits over time. This decreases their inner diameter and stiffens them, which in turn inhibits blood flow and increases blood pressure. In plumbing you can either ream out clogged pipes, dissolve the blockages away with substances like "Liquid-Plumr," or remove bad pipe sections and replace them with a new pipe. Modern medicine approaches atherosclerosis using a variety of surgical procedures and prescription drugs that operate a bit differently.

For instance, hospitals routinely perform coronary bypass surgeries to bypass blocked vascular areas and improve blood flow to the heart. With a coronary bypass operation you create a new pathway to the heart by taking a healthy blood vessel from your leg, chest or arm and connecting it with other arteries to the heart so that the blood bypasses the occluded area. Balloon angioplasty operations attempt to open blocked or narrowed blood vessels by squeezing plaque deposits against the arterial walls, but don't solve the underlying problem of plaque buildup in the first place. Coronary stent insertions are placed within blocked arteries to help keep them open and reestablish the blood flow in clogged blood vessels, but never solve the underlying problem too.

Doctors also prescribe strong pharmaceutical drugs to help patients normalize their high blood pressure, normalize blood sugar levels or lower lipid levels in the blood. Unfortunately, too often the drugs end up suppressing symptoms while the condition they are meant to treat worsens. These medications often produce side effects that are then treated with more medications, and pretty soon you will find some people taking so many medications with unintended interactions that no one can trace harmful side effects back to a specific cause other than taking too many medications. All the while the condition gets worse.

Treating heart disease with strong pharmaceutical medications and procedures such as bypass operations, angioplasty, stenting and expensive tests are some of the most profitable parts of a hospital's business. It would be a financial catastrophe for mainstream medicine if these expensive procedures were replaced by cheaper and safer options you could even do at home to help eliminate a heart condition.

Let's counter these expensive, intrusive procedures with a non-invasive therapy doctors are now starting to recommend, namely enhanced external counterpulsation (EECP) therapy. There are more than 100 studies showing that EECP will safely enhance the alternate pathways by which blood reaches the heart muscle thus negating the need for a bypass operation. By use of this novel therapy alone, patients can often quickly overcome their cardiovascular symptoms and resume active healthy lifestyles.

Are there any other ways to increase the blood flow through your veins and arteries by removing various sorts of blockages? Are there any natural arterial cleansing regimens – an orthomolecular approach - other than the use of cholesterol lowering drugs such as statins?

The basic objective to naturally clear arteries of atherosclerotic plaque accumulations – without using drugs or operations – falls under the principle of detoxification because you are trying to get rid of unwanted substances in the body. The idea that you can clean your arteries of occlusions is sound and there are two basic ways to do so: (1) chelation therapy and (2) the orthomolecular approach of diet and nutritional supplements.

## EDTA Chelation Therapy

As cholesterol accumulates in arterial walls it causes both inflammation and scarring. Plaques then grow from this beginning and slowly narrow the artery's interior to interfere with the flow of blood through it. By the time someone is diagnosed with the calcified plaques of atherosclerosis, usually standard medical therapies cannot reverse the plaques. We should think of the plaques as a problem of detoxification and ask what we can naturally do about them.

Even if you are not diagnosed with atherosclerosis (hardening of the arteries via plaque deposits) and have no symptoms, *The Lancet* (2013) reported that if you are 50 years old you have a high probability of atherosclerosis already present in your arteries. Approximately 82% of men and 68% of women have some degree of atherosclerosis so we should definitely investigate natural ways to strip clean the arteries without having to use medications or surgery.

Just a small increase in the diameter of blood vessels or a small increase in arterial flexibility translates into a huge improvement in blood flow. How can we achieve this? Many years ago holistic physicians discovered that *chelation therapy* can achieve these results and help with atherosclerosis.

Chelation therapy involves a chemical called EDTA (ethylenediaminetetraacetic acid), a type of man-made synthetic amino acid, that is administered via IV drip. As a chelating agent, the EDTA will bind to heavy metals in the body that are stored within arteries and muscles and then flush them out through your kidneys. It even removes heavy metals from your bones!

The EDTA forms a chemical attachment to a metal ion, pulls it off a cell and then carries it from the body. Therefore it can gradually reduce the metal-mineral (including calcium) deposits in any atherosclerotic plaque by dissolving it away. Once that goes, an artery becomes more flexible and with increased flexibility comes greater blood flow.

Ongoing research is still underway, but most results so far are positive including thousands of remarkable testimonials from patients who underwent chelation therapy and eliminated their heart symptoms forever. Holistic medicine physicians have been using IV chelation therapy to successfully treat atherosclerosis for years. Many on waiting lists for cardiac bypass surgery have found they didn't even need the surgery following a series of EDTA treatments.

I have always been struck by the incredible testimonials found everywhere of heart patients who experienced remarkable recoveries after being given EDTA chelation therapy, therefore many years ago I underwent the therapy myself as a preventative. I didn't have any occluded arteries or symptoms of heart disease, but my administering physician said that in several months time I would feel an inexplicable lift of buoyant energy as my arteries became more elastic, and that's exactly what happened.

The reason chelation works is because atherosclerotic plaque contains calcium. The EDTA will bind with the calcium inside arteries and flush it out of the body. Since atherosclerosis is a body-wide disease, if your coronary arteries are occluded then additional arteries located elsewhere in your body (kidneys, liver, lungs, etc.) will also most likely be occluded. Since EDTA chelation operates everywhere, it therefore provides a system-wide benefit whereas angioplasty, stents and cardiac bypass surgery just provide a local benefit that is often reversed in a short period of time. These operations also carry the mortality risk of you dying on the operating table.

Modern medicine started using intravenous EDTA chelation in the 1950s to remove lead and other common heavy metals from the body, so it has long been approved for removing heavy metals (lead, mercury, aluminum and cadmium) from inside people. It wasn't long before physicians discovered it could improve angina and blood pressure. In the years 2006-2007 alone over 111,000 adults used it as a form of holistic medicine. A 1993 meta-analysis of 22,765 patients receiving EDTA chelation for vascular disease also found that 87% of patients showed measureable improvements. A $31 million study also recently found that using it to rid the body of metals could prolong lives. It stimulants bone growth too.

Unfortunately, IV chelation is often too inconvenient for some patients since you must sit 2-3 hours for the IV drip, and it is expensive for some since it isn't covered by most insurance plans even though it often eliminates cardiovascular disease, arterial blockages and high blood pressure. Most people need from five to forty treatments for best results that usually run around $100 per session.

You can also take EDTA orally (products like Bio-Chelat by Detoxpeople.eu or Interfase Plus by Klare Labs) but typically oral EDTA is poorly absorbed meaning that your efforts are largely wasted. The problem is finding an oral EDTA formula with the highest absorption rate. One product, "Formula No. 1 Original Formula" from Golden Pride (available at vitaminsdirect.com), contains oral EDTA and is said to be very effective with a long track record of helping people avoid arterial blockage surgery.

Liposomal EDTA is said to be better than most oral EDTA

products, and reputable brands include LipoPhos EDTA by Allergy Research, Lipo-Health by BioPure or DeToxMax. Liposomal EDTA is EDTA that has been dissolved in lecithin and exposed to ultrasound so that the phosphatidylcholine encapsulates the EDTA molecules. Since lecithin is both water and fat soluble, this makes the lecithin coated EDTA molecules far more absorbable than just the standard oral EDTA.

You can also absorb EDTA rectally through the wall of the colon by using an EDTA suppository, which is a great way of having it reach the bloodstream. With rectal absorption about 95% of EDTA is said to be absorbed by the body whereas only 3-8% is absorbed if EDTA is taken orally. The higher rectal absorption rate is due to the fact that the blood supply in your rectum initially bypasses your liver, so your body starts using it before your liver might destroy it. I've also tried rectal EDTA suppositories and despite people's normal squeamishness didn't find them much of a problem.

The most popular rectal EDTA suppositories are Detoxamin, VitalTox (by Life Vitality/DR Vitamins), Oradix, Medicardium (by Remedylink), College Pharmacy, and ToxDetox. Detoxamin is the brand I have used and seems to be the most popular one in the market.

## Two Orthomolecular Approaches

The orthomolecular approach to arterial health, which means "the right molecules in the right amounts," is another way to start stripping your arteries clean of cholesterol and mineral occlusions. Quite a few orthomolecular protocols have been developed over the years to help strip away cholesterol and plaque from arterial walls, but since they represent a threat to the money flows of the mainstream medical establishment they have not been given much publicity.

One such protocol is to use phosphatidylcholine, Vitalzym and vitamins D, E and K to help remove arterial plaque. For this protocol you would take:

• 1 teaspoon/day (or 3-5 capsules per day, each containing 900 mg) of phosphatidylcholine (Nutrasal PPC), which is made from lecitihin. Lecitihin is often given as a substitute in heart help protocols. Dr. Lester Morrison demonstrated in the 1970s that phosphatidylcholine reduced the accumulation of arterial plaque. He later found that 5,000 mg of supplemental chondroitin sulfate (without glucosamine) also helped with coronary artery disease although 1,500 mg of chondroitin sulfate works as well. Phosphatidylcholine is used as a treatment for atherosclerosis in many European countries, improves cholesterol numbers and treats liver disorders. There are over 1,500 papers or abstracts documenting the usefulness of phosphatidylcholine for cardiovascular disease, liver disease and neurological health. Specifically, phosphatidylcholine increases the critical substance LecithinCholesterolAcylTransferase (LCAT) that transports cholesterol from arterial plaque back to the liver for its metabolic breakdown into bile, thus reversing atherosclerotic plaque formation and narrowing of the arteries. LCAT is poisoned by heavy metals such as lead, mercury and cadmium. Another reason to take phosphatidylcholine is because it increases the liquidity of cholesterol for easier removal. Cholesterol has a much higher melting point than your body temperature but its melting point falls *below body temperature* when lecithin is present, thus helping to loosen plaque so that we can remove it.

- 1 mg of vitamin K (Allergy Research Full Spectrum K) since it reduces arterial calcification by removing the calcium from soft tissues (such as the arteries) and taking it into bones. Without vitamin K calcium deposits everywhere in the body, including the blood vessels and coronary plaque. The calcified portion of plaque is consistently 20% of total plaque volume.
- 2,000-3,000 mg/day of vitamin D in oil form since low vitamin D is associated with increasing arterial calcification and risk of heart disease.
- 2,000 mg of vitamin E per day (up to 5,000 IU/day if you check the blood work). The brand I prefer is A.C. Grace's Ultimate E.
- Vitalzym at 1 capsule twice a day for a few days, then 2 capsules twice a day for a few days, then slowly increase the amount and stop at 3-6 capsules twice a day.

Though many manufacturers produce phosphatidylcholine, I feel that the Nutrasal brand is one of the finest in the world because of its purity. Having visited the offices of many top nutritionists over the years I have also consistently found A.C. Grace Ultimate E on their shelves, which is the only one I would ever personally use for any health condition requiring vitamin E supplementation. A.C. Grace Unique E is triple distilled, all natural, comes in 400 IU capsules, and the normal therapeutic dose is one capsule per 60-80 pounds of body weight.

Yet another even simpler nutritional protocol for stripping away arterial plaque is to use Life Assure by BCN Formulas or PMCaox by Natural Nutraceuticals to slowly reduce arterial plaque accumulations over time. In observing the carotid artery conditions of his patients (which has a good correlation with arterial conditions), Dr. Robert Bard MD has found that the products will reduce 80-90% blockages down to minimal blockage after about a year of use.

Life Assure and PMCaox contain beta-sitosterol that can help stop plaque from forming in arteries and slowly strip away arterial cholesterol. You can accelerate the stripping process by adding a full spectrum vitamin K (Nutricology brand) to this protocol. The results will start to show starting at 6-7 months and last up to two years as long as you continue with the product. These formulas both contain resveratrol and adaptogens which makes them an excellent adjunct for diabetes and anti-aging efforts too.

## An Arginine Nobel Prize Winning Approach

These two approaches show that surgery and prescription drugs are not the only methods that will help cardiovascular diseases such as high blood pressure, atherosclerosis and heart disease. There are natural alternatives, namely arterial cleansing approaches that employ vitamin supplements. In fact, there are several orthomolecular approaches along these lines developed by Nobel Prize winners and other top scientists that we should certainly investigate!

For instance, in 1998 three American pharmacologists (Louis Ignarro, Robert Furchgott and Ferid Murad) won the Nobel Prize in Physiology or Medicine for their research on nitric oxide, which is a signaling molecule for the dilation of blood vessels. Nitric oxide is nature's way of preventing strokes and heart attacks.

One of the winners, Dr. Louis Ignarro, wrote *No More Heart Disease: How Nitric Oxide Can Prevent – Even Reverse – Heart Disease and Stroke* wherein he outlined six key nutrients for heart health: 1-

arginine, l-citrulline, vitamin C, vitamin E, folic acid and alpha lipoic acid. Ignarro pointed out that the key to managing (increasing) blood flow in your arteries are the amino acids l-arginine and l-citrulline that affect nitric oxide production in the body.

Nitric oxide is the body's natural way to protect against cardiovascular disease by keeping blood vessels healthy. Nitric oxide enlarges blood vessels, regulates blood pressure, prevents blood clots that trigger strokes and heart attacks, maintains the normal balance between HDL and LDL (good cholesterol versus bad cholesterol) and prevents the accumulation of plaque in blood vessels. Nitric oxide is the body's way to keep blood vessels free of the plaque that causes stroke.

Both l-arginine and l-citrulline are precursors to nitric oxide in your body, particularly l-arginine. Their presence in the diet or through supplementation can increase arterial blood flow because they modulate nitric oxide production.

There are over 40,000 articles that are generally positive on the usage of l-arginine to reverse atherosclerosis and improve the elasticity of the arterial lining (endothelium). Nitric oxide levels increased by l-arginine widen blood vessels, soften blood vessels (by reversing hardening of the arteries), relax blood vessels (to overcome high blood pressure) and inhibit or melt away plaque, thus preventing and reversing atherosclerosis, coronary artery disease, peripheral artery disease heart attack and stroke.

The therapeutic amount of l-arginine in supplements designed to promote nitric oxide production is thought to be 5 grams along with 1 gram of l-citrulline. There are many l-arginine & l-citrulline combination supplements on the market with the most important ingredient being the l-arginine.

Dr. J. Joseph Prendergast MD also developed a very effective l-arginine regimen that combines 5,000 mg of arginine with 5,000 mg of vitamin D3 to reduce arterial plaque in the body. Prendergast used this strategy to reduce his own arterial plaque and completely reverse his atherosclerosis, and you can find his story on a Youtube video – "Dr Joe Prendergast on L-Arginine."

## The Linus Pauling and Matthias Rath Protocol

Linus Pauling, holder of 48 honorary Ph.D.s and the only

scientist to be awarded two Nobel Prizes, also developed an orthomolecular protocol for reversing atherosclerosis that has nothing to do with nitric oxide. Pauling theorized that too little dietary vitamin C elevates cholesterol levels in the body, including the Lp(a) variant form of cholesterol that causes atherosclerotic narrowing of the arteries. It is not just LDL but lipoproteins, or Lp(a), that are deposited in arterial plaques. Therefore the "detoxification" remedy he developed for eliminating atherosclerosis addresses whatever causes Lp(a) to stick to the walls of arteries and form plaques.

Pauling learned that Lp(a) binds to strands of lysine protruding from blood vessel walls, and thus he stated, "Knowing that lysyl residues are what causes Lp(a) to stick to the wall of the artery and form atherosclerotic plaques, any physical chemist would say at once that to prevent that put the amino acid lysine in the blood to a greater extent than it is normally. You need lysine, it is essential, you have to get about 1 gram a day to keep in protein balance, but we can take lysine, pure lysine, a perfectly non toxic substance as supplements, which puts extra lysine molecules in the blood. They enter into competition with the lysyl residues on the wall of arteries and accordingly count to prevent Lp(a) from being deposited, or even will work to pull it loose and destroy atherosclerotic plaques."[2]

With this understanding, Pauling therefore developed a protocol to reduce atherosclerotic plaque that involves taking vitamin C, l-lysine and l-proline as daily supplements. The reasoning is sound. The lysine and proline are amino acids that act as receptors for Lp(a), and by binding with it they prevent it from sticking to arterial walls.

University of Chicago researchers discovered the proline binding site on Lp(a) that motivated its presence within this protocol. Their discovery meant that Lp(a) has both l-lysine and l-proline receptor sites so you should flood the blood with both amino acids if you don't want Lp(a) to stick to arteries. Dr. Pauling's associate, cardiologist Dr. Matthias Rath MD, therefore recommended proline as an additional binding inhibitor to partner with lysine.

When lysine and proline are added to the diet the receptor sites on lipoproteins such as Lp(a) are covered up, making them less

---

[2] Linus Pauling (from the *Linus Pauling Unified Theory on Heart Disease* video, 1992).

sticky, and the fact that these binding sites are inactivated results in less cholesterol deposition on the arterial wall. They also help to *release* Lp(a) and other atherogenic proteins that have already been deposited within the blood vessels. In other words, both proline and lysine can work to *disintegrate and reverse* Lp(a) plaque deposits at high enough doses.

In 1954 a Canadian, Dr. G. C. Willis, also showed that 500 mg doses of vitamin C three times a day made very substantial improvements in the arterial blockages of heart patients. It reversed atherosclerosis! He also found that arterial blockages inside the eye in the retina were disappearing with extra vitamin C. This is one reason why vitamin C is part of the Pauling/Rath protocol.

Linus Pauling felt that heart disease was actually a manifestation of chronic scurvy[3] (vitamin C deficiency) and that atherosclerotic plaque manifests in order to repair blood vessels damaged by chronic vitamin C deficiency in the vascular wall. Without vitamin C you will have weak collagen in your body, which is something you cannot afford to have in your blood vessels. Interestingly enough, the major building blocks of collagen formation are lysine, proline, vitamin C and glycine, many of which appear in the Pauling protocol for atherosclerosis. The vitamin C in Pauling's protocol does not just help reverse heart disease and reduce arterial blockages but performs other helpful functions in the body as well.

The larger dosages of supplements recommended by Linus Pauling are said to be the key to the success of his "Pauling Protocol." Pauling recommended that every adult should take 3 grams of vitamin C per day (in divided doses) while those at risk for heart disease should take 5-6 grams of vitamin C per day and 2 grams or more of lysine per day (in divided doses) although more may be necessary. A combined Pauling/Rath protocol using more specific quantities is to take 40 milligrams of vitamin C per kilogram (2.2 pounds) of body weight.

The proline quantity in this arterial cleanse protocol is 2-3 grams per day in divided doses. Because it is so valuable, natural vitamin E containing tocotrienols should also be added to this protocol too.

---

[3] Matthias Rath and Linus Pauling, "A Unified Theory of Human Cardiovascular Disease Leading the Way to the Abolition of This Disease as a Cause for Human Mortality" (*Journal of Orthomolecular Medicine*, vol. 7, No. 1, 1992), pp. 5- 12.

Both Solgar and Source Natural make a l-proline and l-lysine combination supplement, A.C. Grace makes a great vitamin E, and many firms make excellent forms of vitamin C (PureWay-C, LivOn Labs Lipo-spheric Vitamin C, Source Naturals Ultimate Ascorbate C-1000, American Nutraceuticals Vitality C, Perque Potent C Guard, etc.) if you want to start using this protocol.

Doctors in this day and age need to learn all the many benefits of the miracle vitamin C, which is practically the safest substance available to a physician because you can take megadoses – and for a very long period of time - without hurting yourself. For our purposes of detoxification you should understand that vitamin C is a wonderful antagonist against chemical and bacterial toxins and even a heavy metal scavenger. It is usually extremely helpful to any health condition as well. Dr. Frederick Robert Klenner[4] said something about vitamin C that has stuck with me ever since I heard it: "Doctors should give vitamin C while pondering the diagnosis." Most of us would get healthier if we took at least 1,000 mg with each meal.

## Reducing Homocysteine

Linus Pauling's approach to atherosclerosis is based on reducing the chances of cholesterol binding to arterial walls by occupying the binding sites on Lp(a). Harvard researcher Kilmer McCully MD found another way to prevent cholesterol from binding to arterial walls, and this was based on the supplementation of certain vitamins in the diet to decrease the levels of an arterial irritant.

McCully found that an amino acid called homocysteine was responsible for damaging arterial walls and causing atherosclerotic lesions. His research linked high homocysteine levels to heart disease, not cholesterol, and showed that homocysteine is damaging if it accumulates in the blood. McCully's research was not welcomed at the time but we now know that high levels of homocysteine in the blood are definitely related to arterial disease as well as kidney failure. In most cases it can easily be lowered to safe levels by taking some common vitamins.

Reminiscent of attacks against the Nobel Prize winner Pauling

---

[4] "Andrew Saul – High Dose Vitamin C Therapy for Major Diseases"

by the mainstream research establishment for promoting vitamin C rather than drugs, McCully found his initial work denounced by fellow scientists. Ostracized, he was banished from prestigious appointments at Harvard University and Massachusetts General Hospital. He was denied a new position for nearly two years due to his research, which contradicted the conventional wisdom that cholesterol and fats were the cause of heart disease. This view was tied to tremendous amounts of money being spent by the giant food and pharmaceutical industries which had invested multi-millions into low cholesterol, low fat projects including cholesterol lowering drugs. Statin drugs to lower cholesterol sell billions per year while the vitamins used in McCully's protocol cost pennies in comparison. Basically, his pathbreaking findings were so different from mainstream thinking that the establishment reacted against him.

Homocysteine becomes elevated in the blood when there is a deficiency of vitamins B6, B12 and folic acid. The way you reduce homocysteine is therefore by taking these vitamins as a supplement, which is especially important as they are usually lost during food processing. Folate, along with vitamins B6 and B12, have been shown in numerous studies to help lower homocysteine levels so most anti-homocysteine formulas will contain these basic ingredients.

Betaine (tri-methyl glycine or TMG), choline, SAMe and NAC (N-acetyl L-cysteine) have also been found helpful. NAC displaces homocysteine from its protein carrier to lower homocysteine levels while SAMe promotes the conversion of homocysteine to cysteine, thereby lowering homocysteine levels. Research also suggests that taurine can produce a significant decline in homocysteine levels too, but frankly you don't need all these extra ingredients if you don't have a major homocysteine problem.

Over the years McCully's theory has obtained a following and studies now ascribe nearly ten percent of heart disease to high homocysteine levels. It is so simple to lower homocysteine using B vitamins (I prefer the Freeda brand) that a regular multivitamin with the right amounts of B vitamins should be added to any cholesterol stripping protocol.

Since you will find the same ingredients repeating over and over again throughout all these protocols it becomes easy to find supplements that carry most of them. The only major ingredient missing is niacin, which studies prove lowers cholesterol (at 1.5-3 grams per day of time-release form) and cardiovascular mortality even with no alteration in the diet.

## The Jacobus Rinse Formula

A final case of nutritional intervention for helping heart disease comes to mind and should be mentioned for documentation's sake and to illustrate some principles of self-treatment. This is the story of Jacobus Rinse. When he was only in his early 50's, Jacobus Rinse was told by his doctors that he had a severe case of cardiovascular disease and only a few years to live. Medicine at the time had nothing to offer him as a cure. A chemist by training, Rinse decided to do an enormous amount of nutritional research to develop a self-help protocol to delay his demise. As a result of this protocol, he lived for over thirty more years.

Rinse told his daughter his protocol which he would mix together and then spread over cereal, or mix with yogurt. His daughter wrote, "It is my understanding that the things that are absolutely essential are lecithin, safflower or sunflower oil and vitamin E. Apparently the lecithin and linoleic acid (from the oil) combine to form the key to dissolving cholesterol deposits and preventing them from forming. When taking the oil, my father said that vitamin E is essential to prevent free-radical formation from oxidation."

The key takeaway is that linoleic acid and lecithin, which we keep finding in other protocols, are though to combine to help dissolve cholesterol deposits and prevent them from forming.

The Rinse protocol ingredients included:

2-3 tbsp soy lecithin granules
1-2 tbsp debittered Brewer's yeast or nutritional yeast
1 tbsp raw wheat germ
1 tbsp brown sugar (or blackstrap molasses or honey)
1 tbsp cold-pressed safflower oil (or sunflower oil)
1/2 tsp bone meal powder (or 500 mg calcium orotate and
500 mg magnesium orotate)

You mix these ingredients together and then sprinkle over cereal, mix with yoghurt or stir into juice. Some people cannot stomach the taste of wheat germ and yeast initially so you can start with lower amounts and increase the amounts gradually. In addition, the following supplements should be taken separately:

1 multi-vitamin and mineral tablet

1,000 mg vitamin C (ascorbic acid or calcium ascorbate)

50 mg vitamin B6

300 mg magnesium orotate, or magnesium oxide, or magnesium hydroxide

50 mg zinc orotate, or zinc gluconate, or 30 mg zinc oxide

200 IU vitamin E (take before bedtime, several hours after a meal).

50 mcg selenium

This formula, developed over fifty years ago, is now called the Rinse Formula and is said to have helped many people safely improve their cardiovascular health. Frankly I think it is too complicated but it does illustrate the principle of combining many different food ingredients into a daily drink or shake, which is what I want you to learn. If you study a lot of nutritional medicine then you can make a similar or even more effective drink on your own.

A popular way of combining the ingredients is to blend them into eight ounces of fresh juice, such as pineapple or orange juice, to start the day. The vitamin capsules required by the protocol are taken separately.

## Heart Health Supplements

While on the topic of cardiovascular disease, let me offer a final helpful note on two of the most important supplements for heart health. These are CoQ10 and magnesium.

CoQ10 is so important for heart health that I need to tell you what I think are the two best brands available - Jarrow Q-Absorb Co-Q10 and Bio-Quinon Pharma Nord CoQ10. Many manufacturers also produce magnesium, which you would expect should have the same quality everywhere, but I personally like AOR Magnesium. Both CoQ10 and magnesium do wonders to help individuals with heart problems.

As a general summary, if we are talking about increasing the blood flow through arteries or stripping away cholesterol the prime supplements might be the following:

Nattokinase – which rids the body of blood clots

L-lysine and l-proline – Linus Pauling/Matthias Rath factors

L-arginine – which can safely trigger arteries to increase in diameter by up to 50%

EDTA – which chelates plaque formations; reverses the effects of calcination (calcium buildup) inside the arteries

Homocysteine factors – vitamins B12, B6 and folic acid lower homocysteine levels and therefore help prevent the clogging of arteries

Vitamins E and C – which are natural chelators themselves

Vitamin K – which chelates arteries

Phosphatidylcholine or lecithin– which strips away plaque, lowers LDL and raises HDL, and the choline within it metabolizes into betaine which lowers homocysteine levels

Many other nutritional substances will reduce plaque formation in the arteries and there are special diets, such as the Pritikin or Ornish diet, that will help reduce atherosclerosis as well but diet isn't the topic within this book of simple detoxification protocols. Furthermore, many special herbs can help with cardiovascular problems such as Dan Shen, a miracle Chinese heart herb that can help remedy atherosclerosis, arrhythmias, thrombosis, angina and coronary disease so wonderfully that it can often replace dangerous pharmaceutical drugs.

The fact is that there are so many natural helpmates available for cardiovascular issues, including atherosclerosis, that what I've given you is just the tip of the ice burg. However, this is the information you need to get started at arterial cleansing.

7
# HEAVY METAL DETOXIFICATION

There is no doubt that we are living in a very toxic, polluted world. In modern life we are constantly inhaling, ingesting and absorbing all sorts of harmful substances that our bodies must detoxify in order to protect our health. One of our greatest risks that has increased over the years is exposure to heavy metals such as lead, cadmium, mercury and arsenic. These metals can bind with our cells and interfere with the functioning of many biochemical processes.

Heavy metals can harm the cells of your body in various ways, but are especially toxic to the human nervous system. Their presence can also interrupt gene expression and interfere with DNA repair mechanisms. They can hurt your cardiovascular and gastrointestinal systems as well as your lungs, kidneys, liver, endocrine glands and bones. Several degenerative diseases are also linked to high levels of heavy metals in the body.

Not to be forgotten, heavy metals also produce a place for invading microorganisms to thrive inside the body. When people are seriously sick you will often find a chronic infection underneath the sickness, and underneath the chronic infection you will often find the presence of toxic heavy metals producing an environment supporting harmful bacteria. Typically it is only after you remove the heavy metals that chronic infections will disappear for good and health can return to normal.

A variety of tests are available for determining the presence of heavy metals in your body and assessing their level of toxicity. This includes hair analysis (ex. Doctors Data Hair Elements Test), nail analysis, urine testing, and blood tests. X-ray fluorescence can also be used to detect some heavy metals in the body such as lead in the bones or cadmium in the kidneys.

The conventional therapies for removing heavy metals include EDTA therapy, D-penicillamine, DMSA (an oral medication for moderate mercury, lead and arsenic toxicity) and DMPS, which is an oral detoxifier for mercury, cadmium and arsenic. If not done properly, using these strong chemical detoxifiers can be dangerous because they can exacerbate your health problems. Other chelators used by physicians include Dimercaprol, Prussian blue, and Deferoxamine.

The holistic medicine therapies for heavy metal detoxification include substances such as glutathione, alpha lipoic acid, N-acetyl-cysteine, glycine, selenium, chlorella, cilantro, modified citrus pectin, vitamin C, vitamin E, folate and garlic. This is just a partial list of the many substances possible to use, but as we shall see in the case of mercury chelation it isn't wise to just ingest a bunch of natural chelators and hope for the best. Improperly done, attempts at chelation can worsen your problems. Furthermore, each chelating agent has an affinity for a different set of metals and it is important to know which metal concentrations are high so that appropriate chelators can be chosen.

## Health Issues Caused by Heavy Metals

Many years ago the *Townsend Letter for Doctors* published a list of 76 known behavioral and functional disorders associated with heavy metal toxicity. In its August/September 2005 issue the *Townsend Letter for Doctors* also listed the signs or symptoms experienced by 1,320 respondents who had been poisoned by toxic metals. Here is the percentage of respondents who had experienced specific symptom:

Unexplained irritability – 73.3%
Constant or frequent periods of depression – 72.0%
Numbness and tingling in the extremities – 67.3%
Frequent nighttime urination – 64.5%
Unexplained chronic fatigue – 63.1%
Cold hands and feet – 62.6%

Bloated feeling most of the time – 60.6%
Difficulty with memory – 58.0%
Sudden, unexplained or unsolicited anger – 55.5%
Constipation on a regular basis – 54.2%
Difficulty in making simple decisions – 54.2%
Tremors or shakes of hands, feet, head, etc. – 52.3%
Twitching of face and other muscles – 52.3%

Some of the more common symptoms of heavy metals include headaches, joint pain, blood pressure problems, fatigue, muscle pain, chronic infections, constipation, abdominal pain, heart problems, nausea and vomiting, brain fog, mood problems and hormonal imbalances. Hyperactive children's behavior can also often be traced to their influences as well. After heavy metal detoxification, many of these symptoms disappear and adults particularly report rapid improvements in their energy level, mental health and mood, the ability to think clearly, and digestive concerns.

The problem of heavy metals is particularly severe and growing because the environment within western industrialized nations is hundreds of times more polluted than in ancient times, and we are absorbing them at a rate that cannot be detoxed. Many toxic metals are entering the food supply due to soils contaminated by pesticides and fertilizers. They are in the air we breathe. We ingest them and they become part of our body, slowly accumulating in numbers until they finally manifest in harm.

Mercury, cadmium, lead, and arsenic are just a few of the heavy metals that have become so environmentally concentrated that they are now found in most everyone. Cadmium exposure results from contact with cigarette smoke and cadmium household products such as electric batteries and solar panels. Lead-based paints, leaded gasoline, exploding ammunition and leaded plumbing pipes can lead to toxic lead exposure. Aluminum exposure results from the usage of antacids, antiperspirants, baking powders, cookware and so forth. Car emissions expose us to arsenic, cadmium, nickel, lead and other contaminants. Eating certain fish or shellfish, along with having mercury amalgams, expose us to mercury.

Mercury is a particularly troublesome heavy metal to have in your body, which is why the government often warns against eating certain types of seafood with high mercury content. Amalgam filings give off mercury, so yes they are also a problem despite what dentists may tell you. However, the removal of mercury-containing amalgam fillings is dangerous if done incorrectly. One of the best books on the dangers of mercury and how it can aggravate or cause inexplicable health problems is *Diagnosis: Mercury* by Jane Marie Hightower. Andrew Cutler has also written *Amalgam Illness, Diagnosis and Treatment*.

Mercury exposure comes from eating shellfish, from dental amalgams, vaccines and the breakage of florescent light bulbs. Many debilitating health problems where doctors encounter "mystery symptoms" (fibromyalgia, chronic fatigue syndrome, depression or anorexia) are actually due to chronic mercury poisoning, but the good news is that it can be removed from the body with the right protocols.

The first step to getting rid of heavy metals is to perform a hair mineral analysis test to see what is present and if the levels indicate a potential toxicity issue. Hair analysis, from a lab like Doctors Data or Great Smokies, can determine which minerals your body is lacking as well as the presence of unsafe levels of heavy metals. Once you know *which* heavy metals are above the safe limits you can develop a protocol tailor made for those problems. Another benefit of a hair analysis before any detoxification program is that you will develop a baseline that you can use to compare results with later on.

## Heavy Metals Detoxification Products

Unless you are using intravenous EDTA chelation, removing heavy metals from your body is usually accomplished by using oral chelating agents. When heavy metals are lodged in your body it will not remove them on its own, so chelators must be used to pull them out and then your body must eliminate them through the kidneys or gastro-intestinal tract.

Of the natural substances previously mentioned, most holistic doctors will use selenium, garlic, cilantro, chlorella, alpha lipoic acid, NAC and glutathione in order to help patients detox heavy metals. There is a problem with this approach as most of these natural chelators are *too weak to chelate the metals properly*. Therefore they sometimes pick them up and then escort them to other sensitive tissues in the body where they drop them off, thus spreading the problem rather than eliminating it. A different problem is that some chelators such as NAC will often pull the metals out of your body too quickly, and this will produce all sorts of uncomfortable reactions.

When people want to chelate heavy metals at home with the least trouble they usually employ heavy metal chelation formulas, and typically ask me which one is best. After years of searching, I have found several chelators that do a good job without causing too many uncomfortable side effects:

Detox-ND or Heavy Metal Nano Detox (PrLabs.com)
PCA-RX (Maxam Nutraceuticals)
NDF (Bioray.com)
Modifilan (Pacific Standard Distributors)
ACZ Nano (Results RNA)

Always start slowly on a heavy metal detox because you don't want any noticeable symptoms. Increase the dosage of products you use only once per week to be sure the higher dosage is okay. If not, reduce the dosage and also engage in some kidney and liver support regimes. Reduce the dosage if it is causing any reactions such as headaches, loose stools, fatigue, skin rashes or the inability to concentrate. Just "feeling ucky" can happen when you start to pull poisons too quickly out of the body, so go slowly.

Since it is often hard to detox heavy metals correctly without causing an exacerbation of problems or a redistribution of the metals, you shouldn't try to do this on your own for what hair analysis or other lab results show are very high accumulations involving the most dangerous metals such as mercury. For this you should rely on the expertise of specialists in detoxification.

Here's why ...

During any detoxification program you are effectively poisoning the body in a light way because you release toxins from the tissues into the bloodstream, and then they can travel freely within the blood. As a result, they might lodge themselves in other areas of the body, including sensitive tissues, if not excreted. If your chelator only weakly bonds with heavy metals then it may not take them all the way into the proper channels of elimination, and then they will be deposited elsewhere. If you dose yourself with a heavy metal chelator in a quantity more than your body can eliminate during a short period of time, you raise the risk of redistributing the heavy metals elsewhere as well.

## Mercury Detoxification

To understand how to detoxify heavy metals correctly we should certainly learn guiding principles from a recognized expert. Lead can easily be removed with megadoses of vitamin C, selenium decreases the toxicity of cadmium while zinc is antagonistic to cadmium, zinc and manganese help bring copper levels down, but for mercury we must reference Ph.D. biochemist Dr. Andy Cutler. The Cutler protocol, which can be found on the internet, is the one I would recommend for individuals trying to eliminate mercury who also have problems with autism, ADHD or vaccination caused troubles.

Dr. Cutler developed a low but frequent dose oral chelation program to help people get rid of mercury in the body after suffering health problems due to his own mercury toxicity. You can find his basic regimen – the "Cutler Lipoic Acid Protocol" - on the internet[5] and in a book he wrote called *Amalgan Illness: Diagnosis and Treatment.*

The Cutler Lipoic Acid Protocol uses over the counter supplements like DMSA and alpha lipoic acid (ALA) in low oral frequent doses to chelate mercury out of the body. The alpha lipoic acid can remove mercury and arsenic from the brain while DMSA assists in the removal of lead and mercury.

These are strong chelation agents that can overload the body and cause major side effects so they cannot be used everyday unless they are used correctly. For his protocol, Cutler takes into account the half life of these chelating agents. This requires that low, frequent doses of ALA and DMSA both be taken so that they can pull heavy metals out of the body *without* risking redistribution of metals after every dose.

Even a *short* synopsis of his protocol involves so many details that it is far too long to be duplicated here, but it can be found at livingnetwork.co.za on the internet. Cutler suggests that mercury detoxification begin with DMPS or DMSA – which can produce very bad reactions *for months* if not used correctly - and only later should

---

[5] www.noamalgam.com and www.livingnetwork.co.za

alpha lipoic acid be added.

Oral chelation protocols for heavy metals should continue for many months, and you must not increase the dosage of chelators too fast to avoid getting in trouble. NAC, for instance, usually works too fast because the dosage professionals use is simply too high. Many professionals I know won't even recommend it. When undergoing a deep detoxification program you have to understand that it will be a 1-2 year effort and that you should not overload your body by trying to help too rapidly. By going slowly and gently you will avoid making your problems worse. This is why I start with a general detox plan of the Nature's Pure Body Program plus Vitalzym plus Kidney-Bladder tea. After your foundation is laid then you can move onto deeper detoxification efforts such as this.

Mercury is the problem child of heavy metal detoxification, which is why oral supplements such as ACZ-Nano, Detox-ND or PCA-RX (which are typically fine for ordinary heavy metal detoxes) may not be enough to rid yourself of severe mercury issues. Cutler has said, "Generally heavy metal detoxification involves an exponential decay in symptoms. For example, half the problems might be resolved in the first 6 months, half the remaining problems (a quarter of the original ones) resolved in the next 6 months, etc. Mercury is the exception to this, with a few months of improvement, several months of worsening, and then slow improvement over many moneys."

As previously stated, using strong substances like ALA, DMPS and DMSA is superior to using substances like chlorella, modified citrus pectin, cilantro, garlic, cysteine, NAC, methionine and glutathione in heavy metal detoxification protocols (when done correctly) because these natural ingredients usually don't bind strongly enough to the heavy metals. By using only natural substances to attack the problem and having no real plan supervised by a professional you risk mobilizing heavy metals from their storage sites and depositing them elsewhere in the body where they can cause other types of damage.

If you use poor binding agents it can be like stirring up a hornet's nest that produces a bigger problem than just leaving things alone. However, if you keep a constant level of chelating agents in the body for a long period of time then it becomes possible for the chelators to escort heavy metals out of the body rather than just stir them around and drop them off in other sensitive tissues.

This is why Cutler therefore recommends doses of ALA be taken every three hours around the clock while DMSA is taken every four hours. If DMPS is used, it is taken every eight hours in the Cutler protocol. It basically starts with taking 12.5 mg or either DMPS or DMSA and you build from there, increasing your dosage by about 50% at appropriate times. You will have to go to the sources to read about his protocol in detail.

At the same time you are taking these substances you should also take vitamin C, magnesium, zinc and vitamin E as supplements to help with the chelation process. Cutler advises that you should never use cilantro or chlorella since they weakly bond with heavy metals and then drop them off elsewhere in the body.

If you are doing a heavy metal detox on your own, the current data shows that it takes from 8 to 10 years to undergo one complete rebuilding of your skeletal system. Since our bones are one of the storage sites for heavy metals we need to take a good chelating agent for a long time in order to pull out many of these substances from the calcium matrix of our bones.

EDTA chelation helps to do this, but a softer route is to use some of the detoxifiers already listed, which will help to counter any inevitable buildup. My preferred list of oral chelators are ACZ Nano, Detox-ND, and PCA-RX, NDF and Modifilan, which I sometimes recommend if there is a history of cancer in the family. ACZ is gentle enough that it can be used twice a day for long periods of time, so most people usually choose this option to get started at gentle heavy metal detoxification.

# 8
## LUNG DETOXIFICATION

In ancient Indian, one of the commonly taught methods for helping to detox the body was to practice daily pranayama techniques, which are breath retention exercises. The theory is that by deeply inhaling clean air into your lungs and lower abdomen, holding it until you can retain it no longer, and next forcibly expelling it, you will push poisons out of your body and thus dramatically improve your health and longevity.

The ancient Indian and Chinese medical schools both felt that holding your breath forces your body to open up the energy meridians within it that lays beneath your body's physical structure as an invisible scaffolding like atomic bonds. Once that energy scaffolding is freed of obstructions because of this forceful technique, the energy within your body will flow more freely.

This improved energy flow, along with the forceful consequences of holding your breath, will help to push out toxins and other obstructions imbedded within your skin and connective tissues. This is why pranayama breath retention techniques often produce skin rashes, itching and other temporary but unpleasant signs of detoxification. They are a form of detoxification therapy.

The technique of holding your breath not only aids in eliminating circulatory obstructions throughout your body, but over time also increases your lung capacity. It balances your breathing which in turn helps improve your health and longevity as well.

Which pranayama method is best to practice for such results?

The *Hatha Yoga Pradīpika* lists several but as with exercise, there is no best one method. Because it is so difficult to motivate yourself to practice pranayama (since no one wants to hold his/her breath for a long period of time and then do this several times in a row), the best one ends up being the one you will bother to practice.

Most people hate pranayama breath retention practices because they can be quite uncomfortable. After all, you have to hold your breath while doing nothing, and in this era of constant mental busyness people don't like trying to sit still doing nothing while remaining uncomfortable. Nevertheless if you learn to do this every day I can promise you remarkable benefits.

The one pranayama technique I most often recommend comes from ancient Tibet and is known as nine-bottled wind practice. It is a technique I practiced myself for many years. The reason I prefer this technique is because it seems to produce better mental clarity and health results than the techniques espoused within most Yoga texts. Three people who regularly practiced this technique had their lung capacity measured, and each told me it had increased that capacity by 20%! I also had a pranayama expert tell me this was the single most powerful method he ever found of the dozens of pranayama exercises he had practiced.

As explained, the purpose of pranayama retention practice is to help open up your energy meridians and expel poisons from your body, increase your lung capacity, make your lungs and respiratory processes more efficient, and improve the energy circulation within your body. Frequent pranayama practice often produces rosy cheeks, brightens the complexion, and seems to also "brighten" or "open" the mind if you learn how to hold your breath long enough.

As to the instructional specifics, the nine-bottled wind practice involves slowly drawing air into your lungs using alternating nostrils. Closing one nostril you fully fill your lungs with as much air as possible by inhaling deeply through the other opened nostril. You then hold the air deeply inside your lungs for as long as possible while staying relaxed (not tensing your muscles but keeping them as relaxed as possible), and quickly expel the air when you can retain it no longer, shooting it out like an arrow. You do this three times for one nostril, three times for the other nostril, and then three times inhaling through both nostrils.

The 9-bottled wind practice steps are as follows:

(1) Sit in an upright position.

(2) Visualize your body becoming as clear as crystal.

(3) Close your mouth and also close your left nostril completely by pressing your left hand's index finger against the left nostril to shut it. Your left arm should be held perpendicular to your body while holding the nostril shut.

(4) Slowly inhale air deeply into your lungs through your right nostril. The inhalation should consist of a long breath that goes inside you as deep as possible. During the inhalation stage, visually imagine that your body becomes filled with a bright light that eliminates any internal obstructions. Continue inhaling as slowly and deeply as possible until you are full and can inhale no longer.

(5) Now relax your body as much as possible while holding your trapped breath within. Hold your breath for as long as possible, but do so using as few muscles as possible. Don't tighten any muscles while holding your breath so that your energy can start opening up all the tiny energy channels in your tissues without having to fight muscular tension.

(6) When you can hold your breath no longer, exhale it as quickly and forcefully as possible through the other open nostril. Forcefully expel the air out of your body using a quick blow out to complete one cycle or round of this exercise.

(7) Repeat this exercise of slow inhalation, long retention, and forceful exhalation two more times. In other words, you perform this retention-exhalation routine a total of three times for the right nostril. All the while the left nostril is kept closed while the active nostril for inhaling and exhaling is the right nostril.

(8) Switch hands, so that the right hand's index finger now pinches shut the right nostril while the left nostril remains open. Your right arm should be held perpendicular to your body while holding the nostril shut.

Inhale through your left nostril following the same instructions as before, hold your breath for as long as possible and then forcefully exhale. Repeat this exercise three times for this side of the body. Thus, six repetitions of this exercise will now have been completed.

(9) When the left and right nostril breathings are both done, extend both your arms as straight as possible while pushing down on your lap, locking your elbows, and lift up your chest. Inhale slowly through both open nostrils, hold your breath within for as long as

possible, and then exhale quickly by shooting the air out from your nostrils when you cannot hold the air inside you any longer. Do this for a total of three times.

Altogether nine inhalations and retentions are performed in this exercise, which gives rise to the name of nine-step bottled wind practice. When practicing this pranayama I always watch a clock with a second hand in order to try to increase the number of seconds I can hold my breath. I mark my progress on a graph that I post on the wall to motivate me to increase my holding time. Most everyone can initially hold their breath for 40 seconds, but after a few weeks it is common for this to become 3-4 minutes.

## Lung Support

If your lung capacity increases this may help with conditions like asthma, emphysema and COPD. Many individuals try to help support their lungs through nutritional supplementation, but it isn't easy. For instance, herbal and vitamin formulations simply cannot get rid of any tar from cigarette smoke that becomes lodged within the lungs.

Traditional Chinese Medicine and Ayurveda offer a variety of herbal lung support formulas, but you must see experienced practitioners of these medical schools to find the one that is right for you. I like Systemic Formulas "L-Lung" for lung support and have seen nattokinase and Vitalzym greatly improve lung conditions when there were blood clots or scarring inside the lung tissues, but in searching over the years for other lung products I haven't found many I can heartily recommend.

Asthma is a breathing problem that seems to be affecting more and more people each year. A famous naturopath once told me that he used alcoholic tincture drops of the little-known herb quebracho – which was once called the "digitalis of the lungs" in America - for all his asthma sufferers. This remedy is so unknown that I simply had to document it for those individuals that might benefit.

Asthma sufferers can also detoxify a home of offending gases or particles using an air purifier. Activated carbon, activated charcoal or ozone generators chemically break down toxic gasses, vapors, and odors in the air within a room. Of these options I prefer the Aranizer brand of ozone generators because of their superior quality and some extra work they do that isn't done by ordinary ozone generators. To use an ozone generator to clear a room of fumes (such as after you painted a room or want to clear it of furniture varnish outgassing) you place it as high as possible in the room (on the top of a shelf for instance) and then turn it on to let the ozone fall down and flood the area.

HEPA filters, on the other hand, remove particles in the air and trap them with filters. There are many reliable quality manufacturers of HEPA filters, which are the most popular type purchased for homes and offices, and because there are many ratings available on the web you don't need any guidance from me on what brands you might buy.

However, I always recommend that asthma sufferers and others with respiratory illness try a Wein brand of ion generator for their home, which can make a great difference in cutting down their suffering. Another potentially useful helpmate you should not overlook is the Wein Minimate AS150MM, which is a personal wearable ion generator for asthma sufferers that uses ionized streams of electrons to destroy pollutant molecules under the nose. You normally would not think that these smaller units work but they have been a godsend to many asthma sufferers.

Several people with lung problems have also told me that they used a Frolov device to help their bronchial asthma and get off steroid inhalers or other medications. Few people know about the Frolov device, which was invented based on the work of Dr. Buteyko of Russia who taught people a way to breath less.

You practice breathing through a Frolov device, which is made of inexpensive plastic, to train your breathing. The Frolov device creates $CO_2$ reuptake, resending part of your exhaled $CO_2$ back into your body when you inhale. This feedback of $CO_2$ causes you to develop more efficient breathing in each and every breathing cycle. The result of training with the device is that with each breath you end up delivering more oxygen more deeply into your body.

The last lung issue we can address in a detoxification fashion concerns sinus problems. For recurrent sinus problems there are two procedures you might try.

The first is an Indian neti pot, which is a yogic method that traditionally uses salt water to clean your upper nostrils. You pour water into the pot, add salt water, and then its shape helps you pour water through one nostril and out the other, thus washing the sinus cavity. The Navage Nose Cleaner nasal care equipment tries to do this for you automatically.

If you use the PurestColloids.com brand of colloidal silver instead of salt water, and wash the sinus cavity with this germ killing silver (you only need a medicine dropper rather than the neti pot), this tends to clear up sinus infections because the silver kills bacteria. Due to a unique manufacturing process the PurestColloids.com brand of colloidal silver (MesoSilver) is the one I prefer since it has the smallest particle size and largest surface area of all such products in the world.

The second modality one might try is a little-known therapy - Dr. Dean Howell's NeuroCranial Restructuring which uses a tiny balloon, inflated within the nostrils, to lift the sphenoid bone of the skull to improve sinus function and breathing. You would have to find a practicing physician for this therapy through the internet and then consult with him or her to see if it might be useful for your personal condition.

# 9
## SKELETAL SUPPORT

Something that always strikes me as admirable is an individual with a fine posture. Whenever someone with a fine posture walks into a room everyone seems to straighten themselves due to their presence. Psychological studies show that there are definite benefits to being taller than others, or simply looking taller because you hold your carriage better.

Unfortunately, most of us did not learn good posture habits when we were children. As adults, the only way to learn good posture habits after years of neglect is to correct your posture through awareness modalities such as Feldenkrais training or the Alexander technique. Then you need to master a continual mindful awareness of your posture (which is usually drummed into children when they are young) so that you can correct it when it is wrong.

The most important thing to do prior to any retraining modalities is fixing the structural alignment of your skeleton through chiropractic or osteopathic adjustments. Once your bones are in proper alignment due to chiropractic adjustments you can work on holding your carriage better.

An old rule of thumb I always teach audiences is that 80% of people in a profession (doctors, accounts, lawyers, chiropractors) are just average in terms of their ability, 20% are above average and of that only 1-3% are exceptional. Therefore it will be difficult to find a chiropractor who is exceptional in skills because you only have a 1-3% chance of doing so. Your chances improve, however, if you know someone who has been to dozens of chiropractors and can therefore recommend one with outstanding rather than ordinary skills.

If you want to fix your posture and skeletal alignment, I *always* recommend visiting a good chiropractor and have seen miracles occur because someone fixed their skeletal alignment. After he or she "cracks your back" so that your skeletal bones are more properly aligned, you can take courses like Feldenkreis or the Alexander technique that teach how to hold your carriage during movement and at rest to improve your posture and bearing. Egoscue postural therapy can also help correct problems as can a number of bodywork modalities too.

When people have back pain, the three major non-medication methods they usually pursue are Yoga, massage and chiropractic adjustments. Chiropractic works quickest, massage results are very short-term and dependent upon the skills of the practitioner, and Yoga produces slow but extremely beneficial results only if you learn the right postures and keep up with a regular exercise routine.

In *The 4-Hour Body* (a great book!) author Tim Ferriss provides very useful information on how to reverse "permanent" muscular injuries and goes into detail about useful but little known bodywork therapies that are little known such as the Egoscue Method, Advanced Muscle-Integration Therapy (AMIT), Active-Release Technique (ART), prolotherapy, and biopuncture.

People often think of acupuncture for eliminating back pain, but having lived in Asia and dealt with many acupuncturists I can say it should have a lower priority than these other options. Before going to an acupuncturist you should try to fix the alignment of your bones and muscles and get them to where they should be to eliminate back pain. Misalignment of your skeletal bones is often what causes the pain and suffering people are feeling.

As also previously mentioned, if you are suffering from muscle sprains you might try using the MedLight 630Pro, which is an inexpensive handheld IR light that provides pain relief for stiff or sore muscles. When you shine infrared (IR) light on an area of the body it increases the local blood circulation to reduce swelling and inflammation. Arnica Montana is a famous homeopathic treatment that helps with sprains, bruising and swelling too.

Popular nutritional supplements developed for bones include Jarrow Bone Up and AOR Advanced Bone Protection with

Strontium. Bone Up is one of the most popular bone builders on the market. The AOR Advanced Bone Protection with Strontium to helps strengthen bones so that the elderly have less fracture risk when they fall. BioSil is a supplement containing silicon and choline for joint, bone and skin health that noticeably strengthens and speeds nail and hair growth.

Many postmenopausal women worry about their bone density since it declines with age. Therefore they take pharmaceutical drugs to treat osteoporosis and osteopenia and sometimes opt for hormone replacement therapy. Unfortunately none of these options work very well and all have unpleasant side effects.

Dr. John Lee MD, an expert in hormone replacement therapy, published a health newsletter for many years in which he pointed out that transdermal progesterone cream did a better job in improving bone mineral density and protecting against fractures than estrogen supplementation or pharmaceutical drugs. Women should investigate this option for building stronger bones.

Other than progesterone, weight-bearing exercise is practically the only other thing that actually increases bone density in older women. All women going through menopause, or about to go through it, should read Lee's articles on the internet about how natural progesterone cream can solve many of the bone density issues.

Because weight-bearing exercise has a multitude of other benefits, it is recommended not just for skeletal support but for health in general.

10
# GETTING STARTED WITH YOUR HOME DETOX

With all this information behind you, it's time to get started on your own detox program. When starting upon a detoxification program you should focus on first detoxifying your liver, kidneys and colon since these are your body's main channels of detoxification and elimination. Only after these channels of detoxification are themselves detoxified and strengthened will your body be able to handle the extra load imposed by stronger detoxification methods.

The list of possible detoxification methods for your body is very long and includes modalities such as chelation therapy, coffee enemas, colonics, clay, infrared saunas, homeopathics, massages, juicing, herbs, foods, supplements and so on. Detoxification is tricky, so you have been introduced to only the general routines for broad spectrum detoxification. Nevertheless the protocols work, and they work fast!

The level of detoxification achieved by broad spectrum applications is what I like to call "coarse dredging" since the methods eliminate lots of poisons without requiring a lot of oversight or causing many uncomfortable side effects. They are generally safe for everyone. Every nutritionist, naturopath or physician has their own experience on detox protocols. I like to go slow but do as much as possible at the beginning without causing any side effects or uncomfortable symptoms, which is why I prefer the coarse dredging options described.

My basic protocol for detoxifying at home therefore includes

Nature's Pure Body Program, Vitalzym and Dr. Richard Schulze's Kidney-Bladder tea. If you just take these three products for three months every year you are well ahead of the crowd and on your way.

Moving to the liver, my basic detoxification routine is to perform a liver-gallbladder flush using the Dr. Richard Schulze Liver/Gallbladder flush liver herbal detox kit. Afterwards I tend to use gentle homeopathic support and drainage formulas to pull out more toxins such as Pekana's apo-Hepat or a support formula like T-8 Liver Terrain by Apex Energetics. Next I progress to a stronger liver detoxification supplement such as the Pure Body Institute Liver Balance Plus, Systemic Formulas "L-Liver" and "Ls-Liver S," or one of the many liver support and cleanse supplements already mentioned. If a cancer patient, I prefer many coffee enemas.

For a strong liver cleanse you need to keep taking these products for about six months. When someone's liver is impaired it usually calls for specific nutrients and detoxifiers that have to be selected based on the situation. That is when glutathione and other strong specialty formulas and modalities come into play. They would be used as appropriate during this six month period.

For the kidneys I like to start with the Dr. Richard Schulze Kidney-Bladder tea or his full K-B detox kit. After this coarse dredging work is done, I prefer gentle drainage formulas such as Pekana's Renelix and support formulas like T-2 Kidney Terrain by Apex Energetics. For stronger kidney detox and support I move onto supplements such as Pure Body Institute Kidney Rescue or Systemic Formulas "K-Kidney" formula.

Most people who want to detoxify their kidneys just use one bag of the kidney-bladder tea and drink a glass of lemon water every day. However, the best liver and kidney support program should last for about six months. You want your organs to work properly so that they can cleanse themselves out and after they are stronger you want to strongly prompt the body's cells to release other poisons. My general routine is to first do an easy, coarse dredging level of detoxification that has few side effects, next support the detox organs so that you can push more poisons through them, and then ramp up the detox efforts after your organs are stronger and detoxification pathways cleared.

For the colon I do a PC123 parasite cleanse every few years. I try to get people who have constipation to do 1-3 colonics in order to clean out any impacted fecal matter on the colon walls as I prefer this to using special drinks and supplements. If someone doesn't have any constipation issues then the Nature's Pure Body Whole Body Program & Colon Program with Vitalzym usually suffices for a colon detox because the Colon Program part of the kit is designed to help with constipation. To heal the stomach and upper gut I usually have people try any pharmaceutical grade l-glutamine or AOR's Gastro Relief.

Many people with cardiovascular disease want to know what they can do for their health. As explained, the powerful supplements include nattokinase, CoQ10, magnesium and special herbs such as Dan Shen. I've provided several protocols that help strip clean the arteries but you should consult a knowledgeable naturopath in order to select which protocol might be best for you. All of them should employ ample doses of vitamin C, vitamin E, vitamin K and phosphatidylcholine using the best brands possible.

As for detoxifying heavy metals from your body, this is a multi-month to multi-year effort but your best start is usually a safe product such as ACZ Nano spray. Detoxifying heavy metals like mercury can be dangerous and requires stronger chelators such as DMPS and DMSA that can produce harmful reactions, so only do so under the guidance of an experienced health care practitioner. EDTA chelation is best but few people can afford it. The rectal or liposomal EDTA supplements are an option, but remember with all these techniques you should measure your progress using hair analysis.

These are all very simple protocols for getting started with a detox program to improve your health. Many detox books are padded with all sorts of information that people will never use, but I prefer to get right to the fewest supplements and protocols, of the many available, that work. Therefore I hope this short list of the most powerful protocols will help.

Every protocol discussed has been a description rather than a prescription because I don't prescribe. I only educate people. As always, if you need more assistance please engage a qualified health practitioner, and don't use any products without checking with your physician who knows your personal condition and the manufacturer who knows usage details.

# Appendix 1
## Optimal Blood Test Ranges

The optimal blood test ranges quoted in this book can trace their origins to those developed after years of research, published and copyrighted by Harry Eidinier, Jr., Ph.D. in *Balancing Body Chemistry*. You can find similar ranges in the works of biochemist and physician Dr. Nick Abrishamian (*Blood Chemistry Report*), Dr. Jack Tipps (*Blood Chemistry and Clinical Nutrition*), Dr. R. M. Cessna (*Multichannel Blood Chemistry and Thyroid Interpretation With Nutritional Assessment*), and others. They are worth their weight in gold to those with hard to diagnose health problems.

Here are the optimal ranges most commonly reported from their work that are found within *Blood Chemistry and CBC Analysis* (Bear Mountain Publishing, Jacksonville: Oregon, 2002, p. 280), by Dick Weatherby and Scott Ferguson, which is a book I highly encourage people to purchase for their home usage:

| | |
|---|---|
| Glucose | 80-100 |
| HgB A1C | 4.1-5.7% |
| BUN | 10-16 |
| Creatinine | 0.8-1.1 |
| Sodium | 135-142 |
| Potassium | 4.0-4.5 |
| Chloride | 100-106 |
| CO2 | 25-30 |
| Anion Gap | 7-12 |
| Uric Acid | 3.5-5.9 male; 3.0-5.5 female |
| Total Protein | 6.9-7.4 |
| Albumin | 4.0-5.0 |
| Calcium | 9.2-10.0 |
| Phosphorus | 3.0-4.0 |
| Gastrin | 45-90 |
| Alk Phosphatase | 70-100 |
| SGOT (AST) | 10-30 |
| SGPT (ALT) | 10-30 |
| LDH | 140-200 |
| Total Bilirubin | 0.1-1.2 (>2.6) |

| | |
|---|---|
| Direct Bilirubin | 0-0.2 (>0.8) |
| Indirect Bilirubin | 0.1-1.0 (>1.8) |
| GGTP | 0-30 |
| CPK | 30-180 |
| Globulin | 2.4-2.8 |
| Alpha 1 Globulin | 0.2-.3 |
| Alpha 2 Globulin | 0.6-.9 |
| Beta Globulin | 0.7-1.0 |
| Gamma Globulin | 1.0-1.5 |
| A/G Ratio | 1.4-2.1 |
| Bun/Creatinine | 10-16 |
| Cholesterol | 150-220 |
| Triglycerides | 70-110 |
| LDL | <120 |
| HDL | >55 |
| Chol/HDL | <4 |
| Total Iron | 50-100 |
| Ferritin | 33-26 males; 10-122 female |
| TIBC | 250-350 |
| TSH | 2.0-4.4 |
| T-3 Uptake | 27-37 |
| T-3 | 100-230 |
| T-4 Thyroxine | 6-12 |
| WBC | 5.0-7.5 |
| RBC | 4.2-4.9 male; 3.9-4.5 female |
| Reticulocytes | 0.5-1 |
| Hemoglobin | 14-15 male; 13.5-14.5 female |
| Hematocrit | 40-48 male; 37-44 female |
| MCV | 82-89.9 |
| MCH | 28-31.9 |
| MCHC | 32-35 |
| Platelets | 150,000-385,000 |
| RDW | <13 |
| Neutrophils | 40-60% |
| Lymphocytes | 24-44% |
| Monocytes | 0-7% |
| Eosinophils | 0-3% |
| Basophils | 0-1% |

# Appendix 2
## World Class Nutritional Vitamin Supplements

Many times people seeking to use vitamin-mineral-herbal supplements ask for opinions about the "best brands" or "best supplements" out there. It is impossible to say "this is the best brand," but many of us do have strong preferences as do I.

Having surveyed countless nutritionists, manufacturers and doctors, I want to share my preferred list that I previously published in *Look Younger, Live Longer*. This is a book I wrote on anti-aging protocols that might be of interest since it combines the best of nutritional theory with the findings of ancient spiritual schools on long life protocols.

This supplement list does not constitute health advice and are not recommendations for treatment, but is simply intended to educationally inform you. Before using any supplements please check with your doctor who knows of your personal health conditions and also check with the supplement's manufacturer for usage instructions.

## Vitamin E

The only vitamin E I would ever recommend to those with health conditions that require vitamin E is the A.C. Grace brand of vitamin E called "Unique E." The only product that the A.C. Grace company manufactures is triple-distilled, all natural vitamin E that is so effective it has been known to heal severe heart problems when the full dosage necessary is taken all at once for the day.

If any medical study shows that vitamin E "works" for a health condition, the results would probably be dramatically improved even more *if this particular brand of vitamin E was the one used in the trial*. If anyone in your family has cardiovascular problems or health conditions requiring vitamin E, this is the brand to consider.

## Vitamin C

Several studies suggest that supplementing with vitamin C at 2 grams/day probably adds four to six years to your life. The problem is which type of vitamin C is best. I will change the type of vitamin C I use as superior new ones are developed and become available in the market but these are my current favorites.

PureWay-C, with lipid metabolites, is a highly absorbable form of vitamin C. LivOn Labs offers an excellent lipo-spheric form of vitamin C. Source Naturals Ultimate Ascorbate C-1000 offers a mineral ascorbate form of vitamin C, which is great for regular use.

Different types of vitamin C are used for different purposes, but the ones used for strengthening arteries and veins should always be accompanied by bioflavonoids, which you can search for on the ingredients list. Source Naturals Ultimate Ascorbate C-1000 satisfies this requirement while PureWay-C is just a pure vitamin C.

## B-Vitamins

B-vitamins are commonly used for any nervous system related conditions such as stress or depression. In fact, the entire vitamin industry was started when people realized that the B-vitamin levels in our foods were plummeting because they start immediately degrading after food is picked on the farm, and too much time passes before the farmer's crop reaches our table.

B-vitamins are very fragile to manufacture and last only hours in the body, meaning you should eat them twice or more per day as a vitamin supplement if you want to receive their maximum benefit. As with other vitamins, you should eat them with food – with the meal. Eat your vitamins in divided doses either with breakfast and dinner so that they are always in the body, or at all three meals if you eat three meals per day.

You can buy B-vitamins from many manufacturers, but an extremely strong consensus points to kosher manufacturer Freeda Vitamins as being at the very top of the list for the highest quality B-vitamin tablets and pills available. This is the preferred brand for pure B-vitamins due to their manufacturing process. Freeda's Ultra Freeda is also a simple multi-vitamin that you might consider as a daily supplement.

If I was interested in the metabolically active forms of B-vitamins such as methylcobalamin for vitamin B-12, pyridoxine HCl and Pyridoxyl-5-Phosphate for vitamin B-6, riboflavin HCl and riboflavin-5-phosphate for vitamin B-2, or even 5-MTHF for folate, many high quality manufacturers can supply a B-Complex supplement with the most biologically available forms of the B-vitamins. However, for the simple forms of vitamin B you can hardly go wrong with Freeda as a manufacturer.

## Minerals

For mineral supplementation, shilajit can be purchased from many different suppliers; it is difficult to determine the best brand although I generally like Jarrow as a low-cost, high quality supplier.

Trace minerals are important for the body, and I like liquid colloidal minerals since they supply minerals in an highly absorbable form, but once again it is difficult to determine a safe and reliable liquid colloidal mineral manufacturer since they often have too high an aluminum content. If you try a liquid colloidal mineral drink and then cannot sleep that night because of the extra energy then you know you definitely need trace mineral supplements in your diet. After a few days of this type of supplementation your body will get used to the extra energy boost.

For individual colloidal minerals such as gold, silver, copper and zinc, PurestColloids makes the smallest colloidal minerals on the planet due to a unique manufacturing process not employed elsewhere in the world. Its liquid colloidal minerals have extremely tiny molecular sizes and thus provide extremely high therapeutic benefit. Available in small bottles or gallon jugs, these are the ones preferred for therapeutic applications.

Other notable mineral brands include Goldstake Minerals and Trace Mineral Research. Kelp tablets are also a way to ingest more minerals from sea vegetable sources.

## Heavy Metals

Countless products are available to help in eliminating heavy metals from the body. Among the best heavy metal detoxifiers are ACZ Nano from Results RNA, Detox-ND (from PrLabs), PCA-RX from Maxam Nutraceuticals, NDF from Bioray and Modifilan algae capsules from Pacific Standard Distributors. Modifilan also has anti-cancer properties.

## Selenium

A superior form of selenium is available as Phytosel, which is natural selenium from hydroponically grown mustard greens. This plant-based selenium seems to be much better absorbed than other forms of selenium.

## Joint Pain

Many people develop joint pain as they get older and try supplement after supplement seeking a solution to their discomfort. They usually run through glucosamine sulfate, chondroitin sulfate, MSM and other products without obtaining relief. For joint pain they might try the very inexpensive Neocell Collagen Type 2 or Jarrow Type 2 Collagen, made of hydrolyzed chicken sternal cartilage, that has been known to reduce it dramatically or stop pain completely in just days.

Neocell Collagen 1 & 3 also works (not just type 2) and I also like Sports Research Pure Collagen Peptides Powder. Collagen is an inexpensive "miracle" product for joint pain issues, particularly knee pain, that might help you avoid surgery.

## Fish Oil

I prefer the Pharmax brand of fish oil capsules, which is the brand the India government has selected to use after carefully studying all the products on the market. This is a brand that gets results whereas cheap fish oil products, purchased at bargain prices, usually do nothing for you because of the low quality. If you are going to buy fish oil, buy the best and get the promised health results rather than cheap stuff that delivers no benefits at all.

If you cannot buy Pharmax then the Carlson fish oil brand is a favorite.

For regular vegetable oils, the Omega brand is one of the few manufacturers that cold presses the oils in darkened rooms to avoid lipid oxidation where the oils spoil before they are even sold.

## Parasites

There are many parasite products in the marketplace which depend on herbal ingredients like Black Walnut, Wormwood, Goldenseal, Oregon Grape Root and cloves. PC 123 (from BCN4Life.com) is one of the best. It was formulated to be safe enough to use 365 days per year and despite a gentle nature seems to work on almost everything – yeast, amoebas, protozoa, worms and everything that causes diarrhea. It is like a broad spectrum anti-microbial, but it doesn't seem to disturb good gut flora and has ingredients that also strengthen the immune function of the gut as it is being used.

Because I travel internationally and eat all sorts of strange foods, every few years I do a parasite detox by using two bottles of this product. I add it to the Nature's Pure Body Whole Body Program plus Colon Program and Vitalzym protocol.

## Mushrooms

Mushroom Science / JHS Natural Products is one of the world's best manufacturers of mushroom supplements and has an excellent immune building supplement called Immune Builder. Hyperimmune egg powder (such as i26) is another immune building product that can be helpful. Another notable immune building product is 4Life Transfer Factor Plus. Epicor is also a useful immune builder.

Madre Labs also makes an immune powder (Immune Punch) that you can readily add to a green powder superfood. In this case, Immune Punch contains Epicor (dried yeast complex), AHCC, and a variety of immune enhancing mushroom extracts. While beneficial, the problem with immune builders of all types is that they don't produce quick results but usually take a few months to kick in.

## Energy

Cardiovascular patients, and in particular those taking statin drugs, often have less energy and are told to take CoQ10. The Jarrow brand of Coenzyme Q10 (Q-absorb) is my preferred brand because the ubiquinol comes directly from the Japanese manufacturer. This form of ubiquinol CoQ10 seems to be more readily absorbed than many other types of CoQ10. Unfortunately, many supplement manufacturers use CoQ10 supplied from low quality Chinese producers whose product quality just doesn't seem to produce the same health benefits.

Normally I would prefer Bio-Quinon Pharma Nord CoQ10 since it is an excellent European manufacturer that I believe is the best possible, but unfortunately its product is not readily available in the U.S. market. Sometimes you can find it available on amazon.com.

All heart conditions are usually signs of energy deficiency and the primary intervention would be CoQ10 (as well as magnesium, such as AOR's CardioMag). Even detox efforts are better accomplished when you take CoQ10 as well.

## Clean Arteries

Speaking of cardiovascular problems, nattokinase is a blood clot-busting miracle supplement that often lowers your blood pressure permanently. Check out the Allergy Research/Nutricology brand (pearl capsules preferred) for a reliable nattokinase product that also comes directly from a high quality Japanese manufacturer. Pharmaceutical drugs offer a better, quicker and more predictable solution to blood clotting issues, but for prevention purposes this is a supplement your doctor should look into.

As to cleaning your arteries of accumulated cholesterol, the many approaches you can try (such as stripping your arteries clean through a combination of vitamin K, vitamin C, vitamin E and PhosChol supplementation) often work, but can lead to buildups again after the supplementation protocol stops. Detoxamin is a form of at-home chelation therapy that contains EDTA available as a rectal suppository.

The Nobel Prize winning work of Ignarro, Furchgott and Murat suggests that arginine and other amino acids may increase nitrous oxide in the arteries and strip them clean, but it seems to either work for you or not suggesting there may be something in an individual that is required for best results along these lines. Even when it works, if you stop using this protocol then the problem often comes back.

Evidence also suggests that arterial plaque, hypertension, and cancer disappear in populations when phytosterols are sufficiently found in the diet. Unfortunately, they have been removed since the time the modern food industry started taking fatty acids and other substances out of foods to prevent them from rotting between the time they leave the farm and arrive at your table.

Phytosterols are found primarily in vegetable sources, and for longevity and good health you should have a preference towards local foods and a fresh organic vegetable-based diet. An approach like CoQ10 with full spectrum vitamin K and high levels of phytosterols (in products like PMCaox or Life Assure) can slowly strip arterial plaques clean starting from six to seven months of usage.

## Sugar Control

There are many approaches to sugar control, which is the natural result of a calorie restriction diet and a key principle to any efforts at life extension and anti-aging.

Under the guidance of a professional, products such as AOR's beneGene (3-carboxy-3-oxopropanoic) can be used for excellent blood sugar regulation. This is the type of product that resets your cellular genetic switches to when you were about twenty-three years old. A combination of Berberine (Thorne Research) and Cinnamon (Pure Encapsulations) is another way to help dramatically lower blood sugar levels. Many other approaches are possible depending on your conditions.

Powerful products containing adaptogens and special co-factors such as Life Assure (BCN Formulas) and PMCaox supply powerful phytosterols that help restore cellular elasticity so that insulin can get into cells. Individuals who first undertake a systematic cleanse – such as by using Nature's Pure Body product, Vitalzym, Kidney-Bladder tea and PC 123 – and then work at a better diet, sugar control and restoring cellular membrane elasticity have a good chance at reversing many health problems.

## EMF Products

TooMuchEMF.com contains a short list of anti-radiation, anti-microwave, anti-dirty electricity and anti-EMF pollution devices that actually work to clean up your office and home. If you have a cell phone, check it out to keep abreast of the latest protections available that will help protect you from developing cancer due to too much careless cell phone usage. Simple things can protect you – learn them. Since silver is likely to increase in price over the years, any silver-based products (clothing or bed canopies) that protect you from EMF might be a good investment sooner rather than later.

## A Simple Anti-Aging Regimen

When people me ask me what fewest products I would personally use for the most powerful anti-aging longevity regimen, I tell them to ponder the following.

Every year I do something for my body in terms of detoxification, and so should you. I personally use at least one bottle of Nature's Pure Body Whole Body Program and Nature's Pure Body Colon Program once per year, along with a bottle of Vitalzym. This cleans the body of many accumulated toxins and you can immediately see the result by the fact your skin becomes noticeably lighter as toxins are eliminated from connective tissues. Of course more complicated protocols are available, but this is the simplest protocol that seems the most helpful for people.

The Pure Body Institute products (Natures Pure Body Program) help cleansing at the cellular level, which frees up the CoQ10 inside cells so that they don't have to be preoccupied with removing cellular wastes. With the extra CoQ10 your cells can then devote their maximal energies to DNA/RNA repair mechanisms. For extra CoQ10 I take Jarrow's QH + PQQ, which is CoQ10 plus PQQ (pyrroloquinoline quinone), a micronutrient that helps stimulate the formation of new mitochondria in our cells. That's a good thing because having extra mitochondria around will help boost your energy and fight illness. You only need about 15/mg PQQ per day. Whenever I can buy it I grab the Bio-Quinon Pharma Nord brand of CoQ10.

Because my diet isn't always what it should be, I would like to be juicing fruits and vegetables but this isn't always possible. Therefore I daily consume a mixture of green powders (phytonutrient-rich plant powders such as Boku Superfoods powder, Rejuvenate Plus, Green Vibrance, Madre Labs Midori Greens, Vitamineral Green, etc.) and red powders (such as Nutricology's ProBerry-Amla) to supply my body with as many different micronutrients as possible that can be used to help support and repair my cells. As a result of this supplementation, I don't need to go through any complicated daily decision process on extra supplements to take. I'm getting my phytochemicals through my foods, through juicing and through these nutrient-rich powders.

Combination products like Paradise Herbs ORAC-Energy Greens and Living Fuel Superberry Ultimate are superfoods that combine herbs together with other vegetables, minerals, vitamins and protein sources for one stop nutritional shopping. To cover your nutritional bases, you basically just choose several of these types of product and switch between them on a daily basis. The juicing of freshly picked, raw vegetables and fruits is a better choice, but since that is inconvenient or costly for most people I mention this solution. These powders can and should be added to juicing whenever possible.

I use Robert Bard's PMCaox to obtain antioxidants, adaptogens and phytosterols that aren't in my diet while a cheaper version with fewer ingredients is Life Assure from BCN Formulas. I also take the BCM-95 full spectrum Curcumin to help manage blood sugar levels, reset genetic switches and help protect against cancer.

The reason most people don't get well by taking supplements is because they are lacking a Core Nutritional Supplementation program. This is key. That core program would include CoQ10 (Bio-Quinon or Jarrow) + Phytosterols (PMCaox or Life Assure) + Curcumin (BCM-95) + Antioxidants (Freeda or Thorne vitamins) + Vitamin C.

B-vitamins degrade over time, so even though superfoods amply supply micronutrients and herbs to help repair RNA/DNA and support other biochemical processes, you might want to supply your body with a good B-vitamin on a daily basis, such as from a company like Freeda. A vitamin-mineral supplement should always be consumed with meals because that will ensure the best absorption.

For multi-vitamins I like the Freeda, Thorne and Super Nutrition brands. For general supplements I prefer the AOR, Jarrow, and Thorne brands. For minerals I use a shilajit supplement.

Basically my formula for health and anti-aging is Food [Organic Juicing + Red/Greens + Nucleotide-rich foods] + Herbs [Curcumin & Resveratrol & Carotenoids & Phytosterols] + Vitamins & Minerals & Biochemical Co-factors [Shilajit + CoQ10 & PQQ + B-vitamins + vitamin C] = greater health and longevity.

I believe this approach provides the best chances for super health and longevity. It addresses the modern scientific and nutritional lines of thinking concerning the many causative theories of aging, and also follows the supplementation and maintenance thoughts of the ancient Taoists and Buddhists who were masters of longevity. If you add the practice of meditation and stretching to this list, and also watch your diet, then this is a simple and pretty complete approach to health and longevity.

If the issue was nutritionally preparing children to have the best bodies for life (or preparing them for super performance in sports or chosen activities such as spiritual cultivation), I would heavily rely on the nutritional advice of the Price Pottenger Foundation. I would also make sure that youngsters had ready access to GMO-free organic fruits and vegetables, free range meats, fresh vegetable and fruit juicing drinks, red powders and green powder drinks, shilajit for minerals, clean vegetable oils and micro-milled lecithin (for the brain and connective tissues), cod liver oil in milk (for beautiful skin) and bone broth soups (to help build strong joints). Children might also take a daily vitamin supplement and of course should avoid food sensitivities and allergenic foods.

By flooding the body with nutrients in the early growth years – making countless nutrients readily available so that the body can pick and choose what it needs – you will give young bodies the greatest chance to avoid vitamin-mineral and nutrient deficiencies and grow in such a way that they express their maximum genetic potential.

# ABOUT THE AUTHOR

Bill Bodri has a Masters degree in Clinical Nutrition, Masters degree in Operations Research and Industrial Engineering, and an MBA from Cornell University as well as a Bachelors degree in Engineering. He is the author of several self-help books including:

- *Super Cancer Fighters*
- *Look Younger, Live Longer*
- *Sport Visualization for the Elite Athlete*
- *Visualization Power*
- *Quick, Fast, Done: Simple Time Management Secrets from Some of History's Greatest Leaders*
- *Move Forward: Powerful Strategies fro Creating Better Outcomes in Life*
- *Breakthrough Strategies of Wall Street Traders: 17 Remarkable Traders Reveal Their Top Performing Investment Strategies*
- *Super Investing*
- *Bankism*
- *Meditation Case Studies*
- *The Little Book of Meditation*
- *Nyasa Yoga*

The author can be contacted for interviews or speeches through wbodri@gmail.com.

Printed in Great Britain
by Amazon